Antonio M. Esquinas
Editor

Respiratory Care in Heliox Therapy Physiology and Technology

Medicine & Health
New York

DOI: https://doi.org/10.52305/JYTN3771

Library of Congress Cataloging-in-Publication Data
ISBN: 979-8-89530-385-6
ISBN: 979-8-89530-519-5

Published by Nova Science Publishers, Inc. † New York

To my wife, Rosario and daughters, Rosana and Alba,
inspiration for my life

Contents

Preface

Heliox therapy book, analyzes the pathophysiological aspects, application methods, patient-ventilator interaction derived from the effects of the application of heliox gas mixture in a wide spectrum of respiratory failure. The health professional can use a practical application guide, update its use in clinical protocols and future indications. We consider that the possibilities in subgroups of patients, selected situations, especially in patients with exacerbated obstructive pathology, facilitate numerous procedures such as aerosol therapy and the effects of noninvasive and invasive mechanical ventilation.

We consider that Heliox therapy is a rationale approach in specific subgroups of patients and selected situations, especially in patients with exacerbated obstructive pulmonary disorders (COPD, Asthma, stridor) and facilitate numerous procedures such as aerosol therapy and the positive effects of noninvasive and invasive mechanical ventilation in critical care.

Antonio M. Esquinas, FNIV, FCCP

Acknowledgments

To Professor Peter Papadakos, MD for his scientific support of this book.

Chapter 1

The Physics of Heliox Gas Therapy

Ahmad Mohammad Alessa*,
Respiratory Therapy Administration, MSc,
RRT-ACCS, RRT-NPS, CPFT, RPFT, RRT-SDS
King Abdullah Medical City, Makkah, Saudi Arabia

Abstract

The primary goal of this chapter was to discuss heliox's physics in gas therapy. To do so, the chapter was reviewed using empirical evidence from many recent studies undertaken on the same topic. The topic of this review is relevant because understanding the physics of heliox gas therapy would determine whether one promotes its continued use or opts for an alternative course.

Various studies recently undertaken on the physics of heliox in gas therapy were reviewed to further the comprehension of this chapter. From the data collected, the emerging themes included the comparison of the physical attributes of helium and other gases. This was necessary because heliox is a combination of helium and oxygen, and the physical traits of helium are the reason for its effectiveness in therapy. The focus areas include density, viscosity, volume, molecular weight, and heat capacity. The reviewed data shows helium rates are higher in these metrics than in most other gases. Thus, it can impact the diffusion of CO_2, heat loss, and other determinants of success in successful therapy. It has been observed that helium has a different impact on the rate of heat loss on the skin than on the respiratory surfaces. Also, being tasteless and odorless makes helium a perfect gas for addressing respiratory issues

* Corresponding Author's Email: Alessa.A@kamc.med.sa

In: Respiratory Care in Heliox Therapy Physiology and Technology
Editor: Antonio M. Esquinas
ISBN: 979-8-89530-385-6

because it implies that heliox has neither taste nor odor. Thus, it does not irritate or create discomfort.
This paper presents a summary of the findings from various studies with the intent of concluding the physics of heliox in gas therapy. One of the primary deductions is that helium is physically better than any other gas used as its replacement. Heliox is presented as a perfect solution to the shortcomings of many gases in addressing respiratory issues.

Keywords: heliox, respiratory surfaces, viscosity, molecular weight

Introduction

Various claims have been made regarding the benefits of heliox since the 1980s, focusing on multiple benefits, including increased tidal volume, gas distribution homogeneity, carbon dioxide elimination, and aerosol delivery improvement. Helium was first discovered in 1868, but it was not until 1934 that helium's relevance in airway obstruction and asthma exacerbation therapy was first described in the context of such an understanding, the physics of heliox gas has become vital, especially when considering its application in gas therapy. The physics of gases has often been an important determinant of how well they are applicable in addressing various healthcare processes. There are multiple ways in which gases are used in medicines. Different aspects, such as chemical components and reactions, have received sufficient focus from medical scholars and professionals. The same applies to heliox, especially concerning how it can be used in therapy. However, understanding the physics of the processes involved is also essential in comprehending the underlying reasons for the arguments made for choosing this gas for treatment [1].

Recent Findings-Summary

Various studies have been undertaken regarding the physics of heliox in therapy. Helium is an ordinary gas at room temperature. However, helium diffuses rapidly because of its low atomic weight. Because of its physical characteristics, one of the core challenges of storing helium is the likeliness of leaking, and it cannot be used with pumps meant for other gases. Table 1 below shows attributes of heliox that should be considered in understanding the use of heliox in therapy. Though not of physical relevance, it should be noted that being biologically inert makes helium non-toxic even when used for an extended period.

Helium has a low molecular weight and density, enabling it to pass through airways and valves with less restriction than most other gases. Its diffusion coefficient allows carbon dioxide to diffuse faster through heliox than oxygen or air. Such is a physical attribute of helium that has made heliox effective for therapy.

Table 1. Chemical and physical characteristics of helium

Physical traits	Chemical Traits
Low molecular weight	Biologically inert
Low molecular density	
High diffusion rate	

To further understand the implication of mixing helium and oxygen to generate heliox used for the care of patients who face respiratory health issues, a study focused on comparing its weight and density to gases that would be used for the same purpose. The outcomes are presented in Table 2.

Table 2. Molecular density and weight of gases for respiratory care

Gas	M	Density 0°C	Density 20°C	Density 37°C
	g/mol	g/m^3	g/m^3	g/m^3
Air	28.96	1292.8	1204.6	1138.5
He	4.00	178.7	166.5	157.4
He 78% O2 22%	10.16	453.6	422.7	399.5
He 70% O2 30%	12.4	533.6	515.8	487.5
He 50% O2 50%	18	803.6	748.7	707.7
N_2	28.01	1250.6	1165.2	1101.3
CO	28.01	1250.4	1165.1	1101.2
O_2	32	1428.5	1331	1258
N_2O	44.01	1964.8	1830.7	1730.3
CO_2	44.01	1964.7	1830.6	1730.2
Xe 35% He 35% O2 30%	56.96	2542.6	2369.1	2239.1
Xe 70% O2 30%	101.51	4531.6	4222.3	3990.7
Xe	131.3	5861.5	5461.4	5161.9

Helium is a mixture of helium and oxygen. One of the most effective ways of understanding the physics of heliox gas therapy is the physics of fluid flow. This is best understood through the Hagen-Poiseuille equation presented in

Figure 1 below. In the equation, V represents the laminar flow, affected by the condition tube's radius (r) and the pressure gradient.ΔP, The gas's viscosity and the conducting tube's length (ℓ). Based on the presented formula, it should be noted that the laminar flow depends on the viscosity but not the density of the fluid. However, it is efficient because the pressure gradient relates to the flow—Figure 1.

$$\dot{V} = (\pi r^4 \Delta \mathrm{P})/(8\eta\ell)$$

Figure 1. Hagen-Poiseuille Equation.

$$\dot{V}^2 = (4\pi r^5 \Delta \mathrm{P})/(\rho\ell)$$

Figure 2. Formula 1.

To further understand the physics of heliox and its application in therapy, one should consider the relationship between laminar and turbulent flow. Laminar flow exceeds turbulent flow in efficiency because the pressure gradient is directly with V^2 when the formula 1 - Figure 2.

In the formula above, ρ represents gas density. It should not be forgotten that turbulent flow depends on density, not viscosity. When there is a turbulent flow, the gas with lower density, which is, in this case, heliox, is beneficial because of the increase in flow or a decrease in the pressure needed to attain a particular flow. According to Dalton's law of partial pressure, the total pressure of heliox is calculated as the sum of the partial pressure for oxygen and the partial pressure for helium.

The Reynolds number is another feature that should be understood when using heliox in therapy. It is the number for determining the probability of a gas developing a turbulent or laminar pattern, which is noted by the formula N°2 -Figure 4.

In the formula above, ρRepresents gas density, r is the radius, while η stands for viscosity. The Reynolds number for a gas is the ratio of its inertial forces (dependent on density but not viscosity) and its viscous forces (dependent on viscosity but not density). Laminar flow happens at a low Reynolds number below 2,000, but viscous forces dominate and experience smooth, constant fluid motion. In contrast, turbulent flow happens under high Reynolds numbers and is characterized by inertial forces, which produce vortices, random eddies, and various flow fluctuations. The transition between turbulent and laminar flow is influenced by flow configuration.

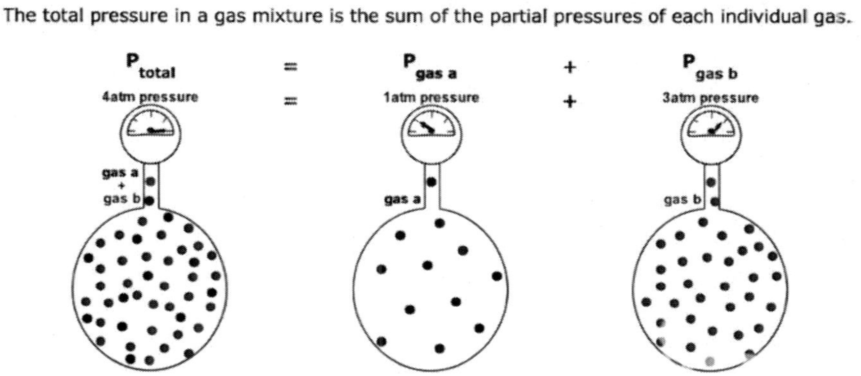

Figure 3. Dalton's Law of Partial Pressures.

$$Re = (\rho v r)/\eta$$

Figure 4. Formula N°2.

The physics of heliox in therapy is also conceived from the perspective of orifice flow. For any gas to flow through an orifice, the flow is affected by density and is weakly dependent on the Reynolds number. Thus, the flow of a gas through an orifice is inversely proportional to a gas's density, as in the case of heliox [2].

Bernoulli's principle also enhances the comprehension of how heliox gas is used in therapy. According to the principle, the pressure required to attain the desired gas flow through a partially obstructed airway can be determined by calculating the difference in velocities in different pressure instances. Bernoulli's principle underpins the understanding that fluid speed is inversely proportional to static pressure.

The use of heliox gas in the therapy can also be understood from the context of thermal conductivity. This is the capacity of a substance to transmit heat. Helium's thermal conductivity is 352 μcal/cm/s/°K. On the other hand, air's thermal conductivity is 58 μcal/cm/s/°K. Helium's high conductivity explains its ability to affect the accuracy of hot-wire flow sensors, such as those used in some ventilators. Heat loss increases when a body is covered by heliox faster than when it is covered by air because air conductance is a significant determinant of how fast the skin loses heat. However, the same does not apply to respiratory heat loss, which depends on heat capacity instead of head conductance. Helium has a higher thermal capacity than air but has fewer molecules because it is less dense than air. Because of that attribute, helium has a lower thermal capacity than air of the same volume. Less heat is lost when breathing in heliox than when the same process occurs with air. Thus, breathing in heliox does not lead to hypothermia. When heliox is administered using a face mask, the face might feel more relaxed than when inhaling air [3, 4].

Helium is both colorless and tasteless. Such a factor makes heliox a perfect gas for therapy because the lack of taste and odor implies that it can be inhaled without making the patients uncomfortable. The physical attributes of helium make heliox perfect for the needs associated with respiratory cases that require therapy. Heliox has also been studied using the lens of mass diffusivity. Diffusion is used to move mass as a result of molecular exchange. Helium has a higher mass diffusivity rate than air and all the other gases used in respiratory healthcare, an indication that the rate of diffusion of heliox is higher than what would be expected of any other mixture with oxygen. Because of such a trait, heliox is considered perfect for respiratory healthcare [5, 6].

Conclusion

Heliox has various physical traits that make it perfect for therapy. Many of these attributes are linked to the physical characteristics of helium gas. Heliox's impact on gas flow results from various physical principles associated with viscosity and density. Such principles can determine its effects on how gas flows into the lungs during various physiologic processes. Such principles can also explain heliox's impact on respiratory care equipment. It does so by decreasing the work involved in breathing and improving how gases are delivered to the lungs [7, 8].

Based on the physical traits of heliox that various scholars have studied, the fact that helium has a low density is vital for the effectiveness of heliox in therapy. The low density facilitates the flow of heliox through obstructed airways, meaning that the patients being addressed do not have to do much work in breathing.

Particular attention should be paid to helium's low molecular weight and density in understanding why its combination with oxygen works so well in respiratory therapy. One of the deductions of the data collected from empirical data is that having low density and molecular weight facilitates heliox's movement through airways. Because of its low density and molecular weight, helium faces fewer restrictions than any alternatives, making heliox perfect for respiratory therapy. The resultant diffusion coefficient implies a faster diffusion of carbon dioxide than it happens through oxygen or air. Such a possibility is exclusive because of the physical determinants of diffusion of gases that have been discussed in various studies: molecular density and weight. Notably, one of them is dependent on the other. Helium's low molecular weight impacts its molecular density, given that one needs to divide the mass by the volume of a substance to determine its density. Conversely, weight is calculated by multiplying a substance's mass by acceleration due to gravity [9].

The Hagen-Poiseuille equation provides a distinct perspective to understanding the physical values of heliox in the context of its viscosity, which is the extent to which a gas or liquid resists the change in shape. However, turbulent flow, an underpinning of heliox's use in therapy, is not dependent on viscosity. Thus, heliox is effectively used to facilitate gas flow under the turbulent flow.

The concept of respiratory heat loss is also vital in understanding the applicability of therapy. For the skin, the heat is supposed to increase faster when one is covered with heliox than when one is covered with air. Using the same concept to understand the impact of heliox on respiratory heat loss might be misleading because the relationship is inverse. In respiratory heat, the less heat capacity a gas has, its heat conductance is more critical. Density emerges as an essential physical value in determining the use of heliox in patients with respiratory issues. Because of the relationship between helium's density and heat capacity, one loses less heat when heliox is used than when using air. This factor plays a vital role in preventing hypothermia. Notably, hypothermia is a condition that is caused by prolonged exposure to cold temperatures.

Because of the physical attributes of heliox, it plays a vital role in facilitating respiratory functions. The primary determinant is the gas's volume, which determines its ability to move and its relationship to heat loss and gain. Unlike what is likely to be assumed, heliox plays a better role in preventing heat loss because of the understood relationship between its density and heat capacity.

Key Messages

1. Heliox's Physical Attributes: Heliox, a mixture of helium and oxygen, possesses physical traits such as low density and molecular weight, enabling it to pass through airways with less restriction than other gases.
2. Diffusion and Gas Flow: Helium's high diffusion rate facilitates the rapid diffusion of carbon dioxide through heliox, making it practical for respiratory therapy. The Hagen-Poiseuille equation helps understand the laminar flow of heliox and its impact on gas delivery to the lungs.
3. Turbulent Flow and Reynolds Number: Heliox's low density contributes to its efficiency in turbulent situations, reducing the pressure needed for gas flow. The Reynolds number determines the likelihood of a gas developing turbulent flow patterns.
4. Bernoulli's Principle: Bernoulli's principle explains how pressure differences influence gas flow through partially obstructed airways, aiding in understanding heliox therapy.
5. Thermal Conductivity: Helium's high thermal conductivity affects heat loss differently on the skin than on respiratory surfaces, preventing hypothermia during therapy.
6. Biological Inertness and Comfort: Helium's lack of taste and odor makes heliox inhalation comfortable for patients, contributing to its suitability for respiratory therapy.
7. Mass Diffusivity: Helium's higher mass diffusivity rate than other gases enhances heliox's diffusion rate, making it ideal for respiratory healthcare.
8. Physical Principles in Therapy: Understanding heliox's physical principles, including viscosity, density, and heat capacity, elucidates its role in improving gas flow, reducing the work of breathing, and preventing heat loss during respiratory therapy.
9. Conclusion: Heliox's physical properties, particularly its low density and molecular weight, make it highly effective for respiratory therapy, providing better gas flow and reducing patient discomfort compared to other gases.

References

[1] Cruz L, Ferreira AR, Coimbra A, Castel-Branco MG. Helium-oxygen mixtures and acute severe asthma. *Allergologia et Immunopathologia* 2009;37(4):216-217.

[2] Hess DR, Fink JB, Venkataraman ST, Kim IK, Myers TR, Tano BD. The history and physics of heliox. *Respiratory Care* 2006;51(6):608-612.

[3] Gianni S, Valsecchi C, Berra L. Therapeutic gases and inhaled anesthetics as adjunctive therapies in critically ill patients. *Seminars in Respiratory and Critical Care Medicine* 2022;43(3):440-452.

[4] Ebeling W, Reinholz H, Röpke G. Equation of state of hydrogen, helium, and solar plasmas. Contributions to Plasma. *Physics* 2021;61(10):e202100085.

[5] Santus P, Radovanovic D, Pecchiari M, Ferrando M, Tursi F, Patella V, Braido F. The relevance of targeting treatment to small airways in asthma and COPD. *Respiratory Car*e 2020;65(9):1392-1412.

[6] D'Angelo E, Pecchiari M, Bellemare F, Cevenini G, Barbini P. Heliox administration in anesthetized rabbits with spontaneous inspiratory flow limitation. *Journal of Applied Physiology* 2021;130(5):1496-1509.

[7] Vanderlaan M, Brumm T. Oxygen sensor errors in helium-air mixtures *Cryogenics* 2021;116:103297.

[8] Jaffe MB, Eisenkraft JB, Orr J. Respiratory gas monitoring. In: Anesthesia Equipment. WB Saunders; 2021:195-217.

[9] Munteanu C, Dogaru G, Rotariu M, Onose G. Therapeutic gases used in balneotherapy and rehabilitation medicine-scientific relevance in the last ten years (2011–2020). Synthetic literature review. *Research Journal* 2021;12(2):111-122.

Chapter 2

Gas Heliox and the Work of Breathing

Ahmad Mohammad Alessa*,
Respiratory Therapy Administration, MSc, RRT-ACCS, RRT-NPS, CPFT, RPFT, RRT-SDS
King Abdullah Medical City, Makkah, Saudi Arabia

Abstract

This chapter primarily covers the work of breath, which is the energy or oxygen required by the respiratory muscles to facilitate sufficient respiration and ventilation. It is based on the understanding that multiple factors underpin the sufficiency of the oxygen inhaled and absorbed into the red blood cells to be distributed to various parts of the body.

The findings from recent studies reveal the multiple associations that impact respiratory health. Some of the studies focused on the process of breathing. The emergent phases include inhalation, absorption of oxygen into the red blood cells, transportation to various parts of the body, exchanging oxygen for carbon dioxide, and how the carbon dioxide, as waste gas, is transported back to the lungs and eventually exhaled. It presents a cycle of action that happens simultaneously to ensure enough oxygen supply to the body and that there is no unhealthy retention of carbon dioxide in the lungs or any part of the body.

From the study, healthy humans are supposed to have average respiratory rates of between 12 and 15 breaths each minute. This is a way of preventing the buildup of carbon dioxide in the lungs. During respiration, elastic and flow-resistive work takes place. Every time the respiration rate decreases, the elastic work increases while the flow-resistive work decreases.

---

* Corresponding Author's Email: Alessa.A@kamc.med.sa

In: Respiratory Care in Heliox Therapy Physiology and Technology
Editor: Antonio M. Esquinas
ISBN: 979-8-89530-385-6

In light of the empirical data collection, the conclusion is that the Work of Breathing comprises the processes through which the respiratory system takes oxygen into the body and ensures that the waste gas, carbon dioxide, is exhaled. Unless someone is unhealthy, breathing is supposed to be seamless. However, when they are not, measures such as heliox therapy can be used to influence aspects such as the rate of oxygen and carbon dioxide absorption to lead to the desired outcomes.

Keywords: exchanging oxygen, absorption, work of breathing, elastic, flow resistive

Introduction

The concept of "work of breathing" refers to the amount of energy or oxygen required by the respiratory muscles to facilitate sufficient respiration and ventilation. The human body's metabolic demands determine the amount of oxygen and energy. This study focuses on the work of breathing in the context of how important it is in the comprehension of heliox therapy [1]. Notably, the appropriateness of Heliox in managing respiratory issues is based on an understanding of how the respiratory system works and what needs to happen for effective breathing to take place. Thus, understanding the "work of breathing" concept is a significant underpinning of how Heliox can increase breathing for patients facing various respiratory health issues [2].

Typically, the breathing process begins with inhalation. When one breathes, their diaphragm contracts and moves upward, as seen in Figure 1. The movement enables the space in the chest cavity and the lungs to enlarge. The muscles between the ribs are vital in the enlargement of the chest cavity during the process [3]. They contract to allow the rib cage to move outward and upward during inhalation. While the lungs expand, the air is inhaled through the nose or mouth. The inhaled air moves down the windpipe or trachea to the lungs. After it passes through the bronchial tubes, the air gets to the alveoli.

One significant aspect that is important in understanding the work of breathing is the number of breaths one takes each minute, which is considered the respiratory rate. In non-exertion situations, humans have an average respiratory rate of between 12 and 15 breaths each minute. The respiratory rate impacts alveolar ventilation, which is how air moves out of and into the alveoli. Alveolar ventilation prevents the buildup of carbon dioxide in the alveoli. Alveolar ventilation can be kept constant in two significant ways. One is increasing the respiratory rate while reducing the air per breath's tidal volume. The second option is decreasing the respiratory rate and increasing the tidal volume per breath. Either way, the intention remains to maintain ventilation. However, the type and amount of work done differ. Respiratory rate and tidal volume are regulated closely whenever the demand for oxygen increases.

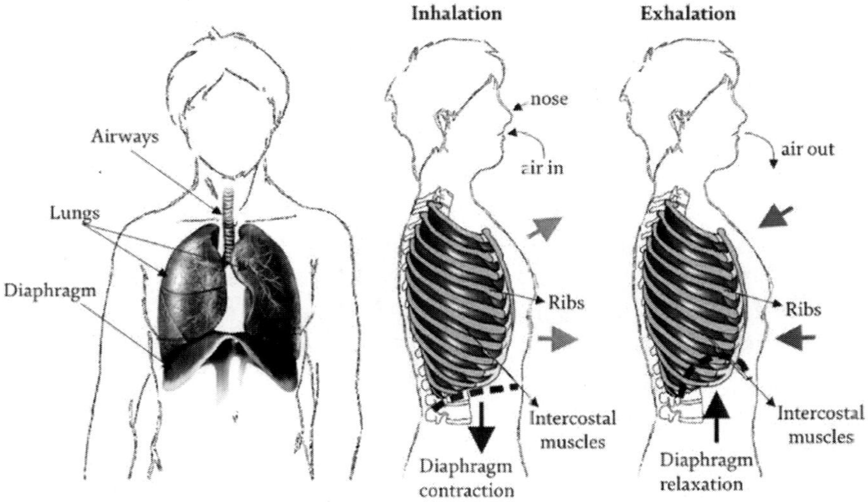

Figure 1. Breathing Process.

Two types of work are undertaken during respiration: elastic and flow-resistive. Flow-resistive work is the work of the tissues in the lungs and alveoli. Elastic work, on the other hand, involves the chest wall, diaphragm, and intercostal muscles [4]. As the respiration rate increases, the airways' low-resistive work experiences a similar effect, while the elastic work has an inverse experience. Every time the respiration rate decreases, the elastic work increases while the flow-resistive work decreases.

Notably, humans breathe in because oxygen in their air is needed in their bloodstream. Thus, multiple studies have focused on the process through which the inhaled oxygen gets to the blood, where it is required. Every time a person breathes in, the oxygen from the inhaled air passes through the alveoli's thin walls into the surrounding capillaries. It is from the capillaries that the red blood cells pick up the oxygen using a protein known as hemoglobin. At this point, there is a simultaneous process through which carbon dioxide, the waste gas carried by the hemoglobin from the body, exchanges places with oxygen. Carbon is the gas that is produced after the body has used up the oxygen [5]. Thus, hemoglobin is vital in transporting oxygen and carbon dioxide into and out of the body.

The pulmonary veins carry the blood with oxygen-rich red blood cells to the left side of the heart. When the oxygenated blood gets to the heart, it is pumped to the rest of the body. At the various parts of the body, the oxygen is transferred from the blood cells to the cells, where it is used to create the energy the body requires to function. Carbon dioxide is produced as a byproduct when the cells use oxygen to produce energy. However, the carbon dioxide must be transported from the various production points and removed from the body [6]. Thus, it is exchanged back to the blood cells that deliver oxygen and is transported back to the point where it is replaced by oxygen that has been inhaled. Once the carbon dioxide is in the bloodstream, it is transported back to the right side of the heart, from where it goes through the pulmonary artery to the lungs. At the lungs, the deoxygenation flows from the capillaries back to the alveoli, where carbon dioxide is exchanged for oxygen and then breathed out.

The process of respiration ends with carbon dioxide being breathed out. When humans exhale, the diaphragm and rib muscles relax. This process reduces the spec in the chest cavity. As the cavity decreases in size, the lungs are deflated like air is released from a balloon when pressed. Because of these processes, carbon dioxide in the lungs is forced out, flowing through the windpipe to the nose and released into the atmosphere. No effort is needed to breathe out unless one has lung complications or engages in physical activity. During exercise, the abdominal muscle contracts, pushing the diaphragm against the lung more than it usually does when the body is still. This leads to an increase in the speed at which air is gone from the lungs.

One area of the work of breathing that has received attention is surfactant, a complex mixture of lipoproteins and phospholipids that reduces the surface tension between the air and alveoli tissue within the alveoli [7]. When the surface tension of the alveolar fluid is lowered, the alveoli's tendency to collapse is reduced. Surfactants play the same role as detergents by lowering surface tension and easing airway inflation. When a small amount of surfactant is applied to the airway tissues, work is needed to inflate the airways. Some babies who are prematurely born do not have sufficient surfactant. Thus, they have respiratory distress syndrome because it requires more than enough effort for their lungs to be inflated. Surfactant also plays a role in preventing the tiny alveoli from collapsing relative to the large alveoli.

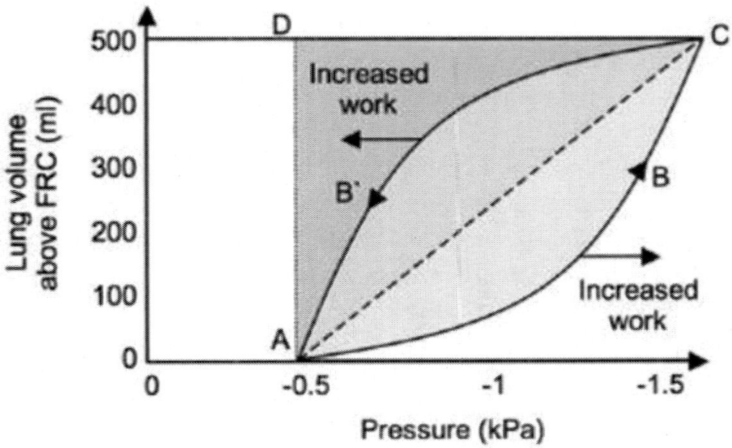

Figure 2. Work of Breathing Graph.

Under normal circumstances, expiration entails using energy stored within the elastic tissue during inspiration. Thus, expiration is considered passive unless the energy needed to overcome airway resistance exceeds what is available. Figure 2 below shows the impact of tissue and airway resistance on the pressure-volume relationship in the chest. Line ABC represents the physiological lines traced during inspiration, while the area ACDA is the work needed to overcome tissue resistance. The area concluded by ABCA is the work done to overcome friction and viscous resistance during inspiration. Line CB'A is the physiological line that represents expiration. The area CB'AC encloses represents the work needed for expiration against airway resistance [8]. When the resistance increases, the curve shifts to the left.

Lung resistance and compliance are essential aspects of breathing work. The gas exchange rates decrease when someone suffers from a pulmonary disease. This phenomenon is attributed to two primary elements: compliance and resistance. Compliance is the extent to which the lungs are elastic. Conversely, resistance is the extent to which obstruction exists in the airways. When either of the two aspects is dramatically changed, breathing is affected. The same applies to the ability to take in oxygen and release carbon dioxide. Thus, the respiratory system might not work as expected.

Perfect examples of restrictive diseases are pulmonary fibrosis and respiratory distress syndrome. Both diseases are characterized by low compliance and stiffness of the airways __. Thus, there is a decrease in compliance as the lung tissues do not bend and move as expected. The two diseases are also known for an increase in intrapleural pressure and the collapsing of the airway when one exhales, leading to the trapping of air in the lungs. Functional or forced vital capacity, which refers to the quantity of air that one can forcibly exhale after taking the deepest breath possible, is much lower for patients suffering from pulmonary fibrosis and respiratory distress syndrome than in perfectly healthy individuals. The time one takes to exhale the air is significantly prolonged for people suffering from such conditions. Thus, such individuals cannot exhale the typical amount of air, as seen in Figure 3. Based on the details presented below, the volume of air exhaled when one is healthy is the highest, while that for one with obstructive disease is the lowest. The volume exhaled by individuals with restrictive diseases is also low. All the volumes, however, stabilize once they reach their peak [8]. The peaks differ for people with normal lungs and those with restrictive and obstructive diseases.

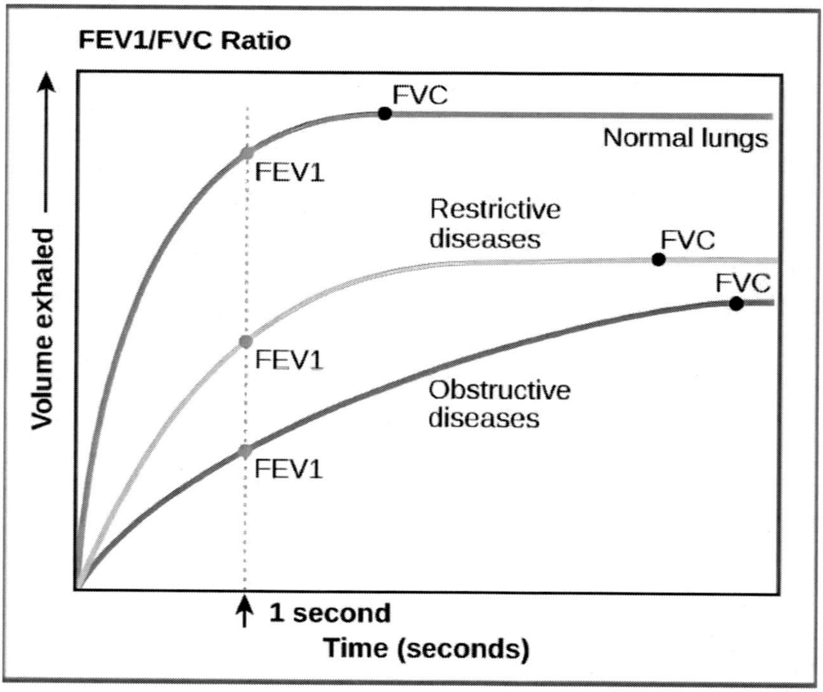

Figure 3. FEV1/FVC ratio.

The Work of Breathing comprises the processes through which the respiratory system takes oxygen into the body and ensures that the waste gas, carbon dioxide, is exhaled. It is characterized by inhaling and exhaling, the process's most evidently seen aspects. The intake of oxygen through the nose of the mouth involves taking air, which comprises oxygen, among other gases. However, only oxygen is needed to produce energy in the body. Thus, the red blood cells absorb oxygen from the inhaled air and distribute it to the rest of the body using hemoglobin.

A healthy human should have an average of 15 to 12 breaths each minute without physical exercise. This is supposed to be maintained so that the alveolar ventilation remains within healthy ranges [9, 10, 13]. Regarding the use of Heliox, the focus should not be on how the oxygen is used in the body but on the factors that determine its movement from when it is inhaled to when it is used. The absorption of oxygen can be impacted by various aspects based on the data reviewed herein. Multiple factors can determine the effective absorption of oxygen into the air and are characterized by the nature of some respiratory system conditions, such as pulmonary fibrosis and respiratory distress syndrome.

Conclusion

The amount of air inhaled or inhaled into the lungs is a significant determinant of whether the blood will get enough air to produce energy. Lung resistance and compliance, for example, highlight the variance in the amount of work needed to exhale and inhale [10, 14, 15]. This results in the variance in the amount of air that is inhaled or exhaled. The respiratory rate impacts alveolar ventilation, which is how air moves out of and into the alveoli. Among the concerns relating to the amount of work needed is the carbon dioxide in the alveoli. This is why air has been moved into and out of the lungs. When a person is suffering from respiratory health conduction, the amount of air might not always be enough to meet the body's energy demand. It highlights the extent to which Heliox is needed to address some respiratory problems, especially regarding its impact on the ability to inhale oxygen and exhale carbon dioxides [16, 17].

Key Messages

1. The work of breathing encompasses the processes involved in oxygen intake and carbon dioxide removal, which are essential for maintaining metabolic balance and overall health.
2. Heliox therapy is significantly influenced by understanding the concept of "work of breathing," which plays a crucial role in managing respiratory issues and improving ventilation efficiency.
3. Factors such as respiratory rate, elastic and flow-resistive work, and gas exchange dynamics are critical determinants of breathing effectiveness and the potential need for interventions like heliox therapy.
4. Surfactant, lung resistance, and compliance are key factors affecting breathing mechanics, particularly in conditions such as pulmonary fibrosis and respiratory distress syndrome.
5. Heliox therapy shows promise in optimizing oxygen absorption and carbon dioxide elimination, particularly in individuals with compromised respiratory function, offering potential benefits in clinical practice.
6. The respiratory rate and alveolar ventilation play crucial roles in maintaining healthy gas exchange, with deviations potentially indicating respiratory dysfunction.
7. Lung resistance and compliance directly influence the effort required for breathing, highlighting their significance in understanding respiratory mechanics and disease pathology.
8. Heliox therapy holds promise as an adjunctive treatment to optimize respiratory efficiency and alleviate breathing difficulties, particularly in conditions characterized by increased airway resistance.
9. Understanding the physiological principles underlying the work of breathing provides valuable insights into the rationale and potential outcomes of heliox therapy in clinical settings.
10. Comprehensive assessment and management of respiratory function, including consideration of factors influencing the work of breathing, are essential for optimizing patient outcomes and quality of life.

References

[1] Cross ME, Plunkett EVE. Work of Breathing. In: Cross TJ, Gideon EA, Morris SJ, Coriell CL, Hubbard CD, Duke JW, eds. *Physics, Pharmacology and Physiology for Anaesthetists: Key Concepts for the FRCA.* 2nd ed. Cambridge: Cambridge University Press; 2014:232-232. doi:10.1017/CBO9781107326200.098.

[2] Cross TJ, Gideon EA, Morris SJ, Coriell CL, Hubbard CD, Duke JW. A comparison of methods used to quantify the work of breathing during exercise. *J Appl Physiol* 2021;131(3):1123-1133.

[3] Cruz L, Ferreira AR, Coimbra A, Castel-Branco MG. Helium-oxygen mixtures and acute severe asthma. *Allergol Immunopathol (Madr)* 2009;37(4):216-217.

[4] D'Angelo E, Pecchiari M, Bellemare F, Cevenini G, Barbini P. Heliox administration in anesthetized rabbits with spontaneous inspiratory flow limitation. *J Appl Physiol* 2021;130(5):1496-1509.

[5] da Costa TD, Vara MDF, Cristino CS, Zanella TZZ, Neto GNN, Nohama P. Breathing monitoring and pattern recognition with wearable sensors. *Wearable Devices-the Big Wave of Innovation* 2019:2019.

[6] Ebeling W, Reinholz H, Röpke G. Equation of state of hydrogen, helium, and solar plasmas. *Contrib Plasma Phys* 2021;61(10):e202100085.

[7] Enciso AE, Fu L, Russell AJ, Matyjaszewski K. A breathing atom-transfer radical polymerization: fully oxygen-tolerant polymerization inspired by aerobic respiration of cells. *Angew Chem Int Ed Engl* 2018;57(4):933-936.

[8] Ganguly K, Carlander U, Garessus EDG, et al., Computational modeling of lung deposition of inhaled particles in chronic obstructive pulmonary disease (COPD) patients: identification of gaps in knowledge and data. *Crit Rev Toxicol* 2019;49(2):160-173.

[9] Gianni S, Valsecchi C, Berra L. Therapeutic Gases and Inhaled Anesthetics as Adjunctive Therapies in Critically Ill Patients. *Semin Respir Crit Care Med* 2022;43(3):440-452.

[10] Hess DR, Fink JB, Venkataraman ST, Kim IK, Myers TR, Tano BD. The history and physics of heliox. *Respir Care* 2006;51(6):608-612.

[11] Jaffe MB, Eisenkraft JB, Orr J. Respiratory Gas Monitoring. In: Jaffe MB, ed. *Anesthesia Equipment.* WB Saunders; 2021:195-217.

[12] Liu H, Wiedman CM, Lovelace-Chandler V, Gong S, Salem Y. Deep Diaphragmatic Breathing—Anatomical and Biomechanical Consideration. *J Holist Nurs* 2023: 08980101221149866.

[13] Munteanu C, Dogaru G, Rotariu M, Onose G. Therapeutic gases used in balneotherapy and rehabilitation medicine-scientific relevance in the last ten years (2011–2020)-Synthetic literature review. *Balneo PRM Res J* 2021;12(2):111-122.

[14] Pleil JD, Wallace MAG, Davis MD, Matty CM. The physics of human breathing: Flow, timing, volume, and pressure parameters for normal, on-demand, and ventilator respiration. *J Breath Res* 2021;15(4):042002.

[15] Santus P, Radovanovic D, Pecchiari M, Ferrando M, Tursi F, Patella V, Braido F. The relevance of targeting treatment to small airways in asthma and COPD. *Respir Care* 2020;65(9):1392-1412.

[16] Sehlmeyer K, Ruwisch J, Roldan N, Lopez-Rodriguez E. Alveolar dynamics and beyond–the importance of surfactant protein c and cholesterol in lung homeostasis and fibrosis. *Front Physiol* 2020;11:386.

[17] Vanderlaan M, Brumm T. Oxygen sensor errors in helium-air mixtures. *Cryogenics* 2021;116:103297.

Chapter 3

Gas Heliox Therapy: Airway Resistance and Lung Volume

Jean-Luc Diehl*, MD

Medical ICU, Hôpital Européen Georges-Pompidou, AP-HP, AP-HP. CUP, Paris, France; Innovative Therapies in Haemostasis, INSERM, Université Paris Cité, Paris, France

Abstract

Helium is an inert gas whose physical properties are very different from those of nitrogen and oxygen. Its main property is a very low density, with a volume mass of 0.18 in a gaseous state at 0°C, contrasting with that of oxygen (1.49) and of nitrogen (1.25). Such properties can favor the transition from turbulent to laminar flow and can also be helpful in flow conditions where linear proportionality exists between the density of the gas and the flow value. Accordingly, heliox therapy has been used for a long time for various medical conditions, both in adults and in the pediatric population. This review details the effects of the gas on pulmonary resistances and volumes, with a special focus on airway resistances and lung volumes. Illustrative clinical studies mainly focus on COPD patients, with little effect of the $He\text{-}O_2$ mixture at rest in stable patients, while physiological benefits were observed in stable patients during high-intensity exercise and in very severe AE-COPD patients with the need for mechanical support. Animal and bench studies are also permitted to extend knowledge about the physiological effects of the mixture. Finally, replicas from imaging studies and of the respiratory system both offer the opportunity to better study the physiological benefits and to personalize the use of $He\text{-}O_2$ mixtures.

* Corresponding Author's Email: jean-luc.diehl@aphp.fr.

In: Respiratory Care in Heliox Therapy Physiology and Technology
Editor: Antonio M. Esquinas
ISBN: 979-8-89530-385-6

Keywords: helium, airway resistance, lung volume, COPD, work of breathing

Introduction

Helium is an inert gas whose physical properties are very different from those of nitrogen and oxygen. Accordingly, heliox therapy has been used for a long time for various medical conditions, both in adults and in the pediatric population. The purpose of this review is to provide a detailed account of the gas's effects on pulmonary resistances and volumes, with a particular emphasis on airway resistances and lung volumes. Accordingly, we will present some recent clinical data obtained both in adults and in children, as well as some bench studies and mathematical models, as well as an animal's model. The presented adult clinical data mainly refer to COPD patients, both in a stable condition and during severe acute exacerbations (AE) with the need for mechanical respiratory support [1].

Main Theoretical Considerations

By definition, resistance is the coefficient of proportionality between the frictional component of the pressure applied to the respiratory system and the respiratory flow. Total respiratory resistance can be separated between airway resistance, lung resistance, and chest wall resistance. Importantly, resistances, and specifically airway resistances, depend on the flow absolute value, the flow regime (turbulent, laminar, etc.), the physical properties of the gas (mainly density and viscosity) and the geometry of the airways.

As compared to oxygen and nitrogen, helium has a very low density, with a volume mass of 0.18 in a gaseous state at 0°C, contrasting with that of oxygen (1.49) and of nitrogen (1.25). Such a low density can induce benefits with regard to airway resistance.

1. A transition from turbulent to laminar flow is expected to occur more proximally in the airways, reducing inspiratory and expiratory resistances. Despite its simplicity, the perfect pipe model provides a useful comparison, indicating that the transition from turbulent to laminar flow occurs when Reynold's number (Re) drops below the 2000 limit. Re is calculated as: (V.D.d) / η; where V is the mean linear

velocity, D is the pipe's diameter, d the fluid's density, and η the dynamic viscosity of the fluid.

2. In airways where flow remains turbulent, an additional benefit can also be expected considering the linear proportionality between the density of the gas and the flow value.

However, helium's viscosity is 14% higher than that of nitrogen. Based on Poiseuille's law, the resistance in a perfect pipe is equal to (8.l. η) / ($\Pi.r^4$), where l is the pipe's length, η is its viscosity, and r is its radius. This can cause an increase in respiratory resistance in cases of pure laminar flow.

Altogether, there is nevertheless a strong case for using heliox in some clinical situations characterized by airway obstruction, anticipating a global fall in respiratory resistances with potentially clinical benefits:

1. Diminution in the resistive inspiratory work of breathing
2. Facilitation of lung expiratory emptying leads to less dynamic hyperinflation, therefore diminishing elastic inspiratory work of breathing and putting diaphragm in a more favorable geometric configuration

However, one should keep in mind that the airway network is characterized by its great complexity, with numerous series (23 generations) of branching tubes becoming narrower, shorter, and more numerous as they are located deeper in the lungs. Moreover, there are great variations in the lung's pathologic processes in the clinical setting, so that the prediction of the heliox's effects on respiratory resistances and volumes is not so easy to perform. Additionally, the entrance condition is of great importance since disturbance and/or turbulence can be carried downstream in the airways. Finally, changes in flow values and profiles can have a significant impact on resistances. However, fortunately, we can refer to classical and recent clinical, animal, and bench studies, aiming to more precisely detail these effects [2].

Clinical Studies: COPD

Stable COPD at Rest and During Exercise

Laveneziana et al., performed a nice physiological study in 11 stable COPD patients breathing either room air or Heliox (79% He – 21% O_2) both at rest and during high-intensity exercise [1]. While end-expiratory lung volume remained unchanged while breathing Heliox at rest, they observed a significant decrease of 0.23 L during exercise, in addition to improvements in indices of cardio-circulatory function. The authors hypothesized reduced expiratory resistances, a slower breathing pattern, and an increase in maximal flow-volume envelope as reasons for end-expiratory lung volume improvement while breathing Heliox. This study emphasizes the importance of flow conditions in determining the effect of Heliox on stable COPD patients.

Such results are in accordance with a study from Pecchiari et al., performed on 22 stable COPD patients, most of whom exhibited expiratory flow limitation either in the sitting position (n=13) or in the supine position (n=18) [2]. Heliox was tested, and the authors concluded that the mixture had no effect on dynamic hyperinflation, but it is important to note that the patients were studied only at rest and not during exercise.

To increase clarity, replace with: Finally, Palange et al., looked at how Heliox (79% He and 21% O2) affected the ability of 12 stable COPD patients to do exercise for long periods of time. They also reported a significant reduction in lung dynamic hyperinflation, in a range comparable to that reported by Laveneziana et al., [3]. The authors did not observe such a benefit at rest while breathing Heliox, in line with the results reported by Laveneziana et al., and by Pecchiari et al., [2].

Severe AE-COPD Patients Under Invasive Mechanical Ventilation

Tassaux et al., studied 23 COPD patients shortly after tracheal intubation [4]. The most frequent reason for intubation was acute exacerbations. They compared 3 periods with air-O_2, He-O, and again air-O_2 (permitting to assess stability), keeping the FiO_2 constant (range 0.21 to 0.40). They mostly reported a significant improvement in intrinsic PEEP and trapped volume while breathing the He-O2 mixture, suggesting an improvement in expiratory resistances. They also reported unmodified respiratory system compliance and a significant decrease in peak value, indicating an improvement in inspiratory resistance. Additionally, the authors used a test lung model, with results in accordance with the clinical study.

The same group confirmed and extended these results in a study of 10 COPD patients studied early after intubation at different external PEEP levels and using the multiple inert gas elimination technique (MIGET) [5]. They observed that external PEEP and the He-O_2 mixture comparably reduced intrinsic PEEP and the trapped volume, while He-O_2 reduced in addition inspiratory resistances without significant modification in the ventilation/perfusion profile as assessed by MIGET. Interestingly, external PEEP and the He-O2 mixture had cumulatively favorable effects.

Diehl et al., studied 13 severe AE-COPD patients under invasive mechanical ventilation [6]. Patients were evaluated just before extubation in all patients and after extubation in five patients, while the patients were spontaneously breathing without mechanical assistance. Patients were breathing either He-O_2 or air-O_2 mixtures in a randomized order. FiO_2 was kept constant between the 2 periods. The He-O2 period was associated with a statistically significant 31% reduction in breathing work, mostly due to a reduction in its resistive component, while a moderate reduction in the dynamic intrinsic PEEP was also observed. Similar results were observed after extubation. The breathing pattern was not modified.

The same authors also studied a different group of 13 AE-COPD patients, using the same design as in the study from Tassaux et al., [4,7]. Globally, similar results were observed, although there was a less pronounced reduction in static intrinsic PEEP. In addition, the static intrinsicddynamic intrinsic PEEP ratio was quantified, as was the difference between the airway pressure observed during an inspiratory pause at the point of zero flow and the airway pressure after 5 seconds of occlusion. No significant difference was observed between the 2 periods (air-O_2 and He-O_2) for these parameters, considered good indicators of pendelluft and stress relaxation phenomena implicated in lung heterogeneities of ventilation. The authors concluded that the helium-oxygen mixture has little influence on ventilation heterogeneity.

COPD patients: Synthesis. Based on the previously mentioned studies, Table 1 synthesizes the effects of Heliox on respiratory resistance and volumes in COPD patients under different conditions. While no major effect was observed at rest, benefits were observed at high-intensity exercise and during very severe exacerbations during the ICU-course.

Table 1. Effects of Heliox in COPD patients, according to different physical or medical conditions

condition	Stable COPD at rest			Stable COPD during exercise		AE-COPD under IMV, passive patients			AE-COPD, IMV weaning, spontaneously breathing
Study	Laveneziana (1)	Pecchiari (2)	Palange (3)	Laveneziana (1)	Palange (3)	Tassaux (4)	Jolliet (5)	Diehl (7)	Diehl (6)
Airway Inspiratory resistances	-	-	-	-	-	+	+	+	+
Airway Expiratory resistances	-	-	-	+	+	+	+	+	+
Lung volume	-	-	-	+	+	+	+	+	+

- Indicates a lack of benefit on the corresponding parameter; + indicates a benefit on the corresponding parameter.

Clinical Studies: Pediatrics

Del Puppo et al., presented an original retrospective study based on CT scans of 14 children suffering from congenital laryngotracheal stenosis and one control [8]. Congenital laryngotracheal stenosis is a rare clinical condition in which heliox therapy could be an interesting therapeutic option. They performed 3D reconstructions of laryngotracheal stenosis, which were used for volumetric generation and modulation of fluid flows. Fluid flow computations were used for four mixtures: air and He-O2 with helium fractions of 80%, 70%, and 60%. Pressure drops and resistances decreased significantly between Air and Heliox 80, with an apparent more pronounced effect in the more severe stenoses. Despite some limitations of the model, it presents arguments for the use of the mixture in more severe cases.

In line with this study, Paxman et al., presented an experimental evaluation of pressure drop for air flows and Heliox flows in upper and central airway replicas of young children [9]. Such an approach is very interesting since turbulence generated upstream can influence flow patterns downstream in the trachea and bronchi, which was rather confirmed by the authors, allowing them to propose an airway resistance model.

Diferences between Men and Women

While lung elasticity is similar between females and males, there is strong evidence of lower airway sizes in females. Mann et al., studied 9 healthy women and 9 healthy men of the same age during high-intensity exercises performed either while breathing air or Heliox [10]. For both sexes, heliox breathing was associated with a reduction in work of breathing (Campbell's method), principally due to reductions in resistive work with an indication of a predominant diminution in turbulent resistances. Plotting the work of breathing against minute ventilation during exercise, women breathing Heliox had a similar relationship to men breathing room air.

Animal Study

D'Angelo et al., recently investigated the effects of Heliox in an animal model of obstructive apnea-hypopnea syndrome [11]. Twenty-two rabbits were anesthetized and studied while spontaneously breathing with tidal inspiratory flow limitation. Heliox increased peak inspiratory flow, but no animal eliminated inspiratory flow limitation, contrary to C-PAP 6 cmH_2O. Benefits in flow varied notably between animals, allowing the authors to classify them as responders and non-responders. Modulization of the upper airways as a non-linear resistor with different pressure-volume curves, lengths, and diameters was useful to simulate the different effects of Heliox in animals, illustrating the importance of mechanical and geometrical factors.

Bench Studies

Katz et al., published in 2011 focusing on the effects of heterogeneous airway obstructions on the distribution of air and Heliox [12]. Based on a 2-compartment (of different resistances and identical compliance) adult test lung, they observed a more uniform distribution with Heliox as well as an increase in the delivered gas volume. They also performed an engineering analysis illustrating the benefit of heliox on density-dependent resistances.

Katz et al., performed a numerical study of mechanical ventilation in newborns, a condition where mechanical ventilation can be particularly challenging mainly because of the small airway dimensions [13]. They assessed the effects of different medical gas mixtures and reported that the low-density Heliox provided a wider margin of safety than the other gas mixtures. Due to its high density, the Xenon mixture was the most deleterious for airway resistance [14].

Martin et al., performed a nice bench study comparing simulated inspiratory efforts with He-O_2 (78/22 and 65/35 %) or Air-O_2, with various obstructive disease patterns, and with or without pressure support [15]. They observed the lowest inspiratory effort for the He-O_2 mixtures using parabolic resistors, while little effect was observed for linear resistances, less influenced by the density of the mixture. Reductions in inspiratory efforts were cumulative between helium mixtures and the different levels of pressure support.

The same group also performed bench experiments focusing on expiratory time constants measured using a 2-compartment mechanical test lung mimicking heterogeneous airway obstruction [15]. A mathematical model was also employed. In this model, expiratory time constants were reduced by substituting He-O_2 in place of air-O_2. The authors also reported important limitations of time constants reported at the ventilator level.

Key Messages

1. Strong evidence supports the benefit of He-O2 mixtures for lowering inspiratory resistance in severe obstructive airway diseases.
2. Strong evidence supports the benefit of He-O2 mixtures for lowering expiratory resistance in severe obstructive airway diseases, therefore limiting dynamic hyperinflation.
3. Most of the recent clinical studies focused on COPD patients, without clear benefit at rest in stable patients, contrasting with stable patients during high-intensity exercise and very severe AE-COPD patients with the need for mechanical support.
4. Replica from imaging studies offer the opportunity to better study the physiological benefits of He-O2 mixtures.
5. Modulization of the respiratory system also offers the opportunity to better study the physiological benefits of He-O2 mixtures.

Conclusion

During the last twenty years, a significant amount of bench, clinical, and animal studies has permitted us to better delineate the benefits and limits of Heliox therapy on respiratory resistances and volumes. Accordingly, the best clinical results were observed in stable COPD patients during exercise and mainly in severe AE-COPD patients under mechanical ventilation. As a perspective, both airways replica based on imaging studies and modelization of the respiratory system in normal and pathological conditions could strengthen our general knowledge and help predict an individual benefit of Heliox therapy. This could be of paramount importance for a personalized approach.

References

[1] Laveneziana P, Valli G, Onorati P, Paoletti P, Ferrazza AM, Palange P. Effect of heliox on heart rate kinetics and dynamic hyperinflation during high-intensity exercise in COPD. *Eur J Appl Physiol* 2011;111(2):225-34.

[2] Pecchiari M, Pelucchi A, D'Angelo E, Foresi A, Milic-Emili J, D'Angelo E. Effect of Heliox Breathing on Dynamic Hyperinflation in COPD Patients. *Chest* 2004 ;125(6) :2075-82.

[3] Palange P, Valli G, Onorati P, Antonucci R, Paoletti P, Rosato A, et al., Effect of heliox on lung dynamic hyperinflation, dyspnea, and exercise endurance capacity in COPD patients. *Journal of Applied Physiology* 2004;97(5):1637-42.

[4] Tassaux D, Jolliet P, Roeseler J, Chevrolet JC. Effects of helium-oxygen on intrinsic positive end-expiratory pressure in intubated and mechanically ventilated patients with severe chronic obstructive pulmonary disease. *Critical Care Medicine* 2000 ;28(8) :2721-8.

[5] Jolliet P, Watremez C, Roeseler J, Ngengiyumva JC, De Kock M, Clerbaux T, et al., Comparative effects of helium-oxygen and external positive end-expiratory pressure on respiratory mechanics, gas exchange, and ventilation-perfusion relationships in mechanically ventilated patients with chronic obstructive pulmonary disease. *Intensive Care Med* 2003;29(9):1442-50.

[6] Diehl JL, Mercat A, Guérot E, Aïssa F, Teboul JL, Richard C, et al., Helium/oxygen mixture reduces the work of breathing at the end of the weaning process in patients with severe chronic obstructive pulmonary disease: *Critical Care Medicine* 2003;31(5):1415-20.

[7] Diehl JL, Peigne V, Guérot E, Faisy C, Lecourt L, Mercat A. Helium in the adult critical care setting. *Ann Intensive Care* 2011;1(1):24.

[8] Del Puppo M, Meister L, Médale M, Allary C, Nicollas R, Moreddu E. Heliox simulations for initial management of congenital laryngotracheal stenosis. *Pediatric Pulmonology* 2023;58(1):230-8.

[9] Paxman T, Noga M, Finlay WH, Martin AR. Experimental evaluation of pressure drop for flows of air and heliox through upper and central conducting airway replicas of 4- to 8-year-old children. *Journal of Biomechanics* 2019;82:134-41.

[10] Mann LM, Granger EA, Chan JS, Yu A, Molgat-Seon Y, Dominelli PB. Minimizing airflow turbulence in women lowers the work of breathing to levels similar to men. *Journal of Applied Physiology* 2020;129 (2):410-8.

[11] d'Angelo E, Pecchiari M, Bellemare F, Cevenini G, Barbini P. Heliox administration in anesthetized rabbits with spontaneous inspiratory flow limitation. *Journal of Applied Physiology* 2021;130(5):1496-509.

[12] Katz IM, Martin AR, Muller PA, Terzibachi K, Feng CH, Caillibotte G, et al., The ventilation distribution of helium–oxygen mixtures and the role of inertial losses in the presence of heterogeneous airway obstructions. *Journal of Biomechanics* 2011;44(6):1137-43.

[13] Katz I, Milet A, Chalopin M, Farjot G. Numerical analysis of mechanical ventilation using high-concentration medical gas mixtures in newborns. *Med Gas Res* 2019;9(4):213.

[14] Martin AR, Katz IM, Jenöfi K, Caillibotte G, Brochard L, Texereau J. Bench experiments comparing simulated inspiratory effort when breathing helium-oxygen mixtures to that during positive pressure support with air. *BMC Pulm Med* 2012;12(1):62.

[15] Martin AR, Katz IM, Terzibachi K, Gouinaud L, Caillibotte G, Texereau J. Bench and mathematical modeling of the effects of breathing a helium/oxygen mixture on expiratory time constants in the presence of heterogeneous airway obstructions. *BioMed Eng OnLine* 2012;11(1):27.

Chapter 4

Gas Exchange and Heliox

Kishore Kumar[1,*], BSc, MSc, PhD, FNIV
Kumari Sulochana[2], BSc, MSc, PhD, FNIV
Manigandan Venkatesan[3], BSc, MSc, MTech, FNIV
and Antonio M. Esquinas[4], MD, PhD, FCCP

[1]Department of Respiratory Therapy, College of Pharmacy and Applied Medical Science, Dar Al Uloom University, Riyadh, Saudi Arabia
[2]Division of Respiratory Therapy, Bharti Hospital and Research Centre, Pune, India
[3]Department of Medicine, University of Texas Health Science Centre, San Antonio, Texas, USA
[4]Intensive Care Unit, Hospital Morales Meseguer Molina Segura, Murcia, Spain

Abstract

Gas exchange plays a fundamental role in respiratory physiology, with efficient ventilation and perfusion crucial for maintaining optimal oxygenation and carbon dioxide elimination. Heliox therapy, a mixture of helium and oxygen, has emerged as a promising intervention for respiratory conditions characterized by airway obstruction. By capitalizing on helium's unique physical properties, including reduced density and improved flow dynamics, heliox therapy aims to alleviate airway resistance and decrease the work of breathing. Clinical studies investigating the efficacy of heliox therapy in conditions such as asthma, chronic obstructive pulmonary disease (COPD), and upper airway obstruction are reviewed, highlighting its potential to improve gas exchange and enhance respiratory function.

* Corresponding Author's Email: cmkishorekumar17@gmail.com

In: Respiratory Care in Heliox Therapy Physiology and Technology
Editor: Antonio M. Esquinas
ISBN: 979-8-89530-385-6

Keywords: gas exchange, ventilation, heliox, exchange, helium-oxygen

Introduction

The primary role of the lungs is to facilitate ventilation and provide a site for the exchange of carbon dioxide and oxygen. Ventilation is the process of gases flowing into and out of the lungs. This mechanism permits oxygen (O_2) to enter the body via the alveoli, transferring into the bloodstream while simultaneously facilitating the elimination of carbon dioxide (CO_2) from the bloodstream through the alveoli. The human body requires oxygen to pass through the lungs, enter the circulatory system, and ultimately reach the tissues to provide a continuous oxygen supply.

Normally, this mechanism is well integrated; however, in diseased conditions, impaired gas exchange can alter physiologic balance which threaten survival. Oxygen is vital for sustaining life, and inadequate oxygen levels in the tissues, known as hypoxia, can lead to cellular damage in critical organs like the heart and brain. CO_2, a metabolic byproduct, needs to be eliminated from the body. Accumulation of CO_2, often caused by inadequate breathing (alveolar hypoventilation), leads to a drop in pH (acidosis). Conversely, excessive removal of CO_2 from the body through hyperventilation (alveolar hyperventilation) raises pH levels, causing alkalosis [1].

The lungs consist of approximately 300 million alveoli, which are tiny polyhedrons filled with gas (O_2 and CO_2). These alveoli have thin walls supported by a network of capillaries and a minimal interstitial matrix. Each alveolus expands during inhalation, becoming rich in O_2 and low in CO_2, which passes down from the bronchial tree. Upon exhalation, the alveoli contract, expelling gas that is high in CO_2 and low in O_2 through the mouth. This process, known as ventilation, facilitates the exchange of gases. The capillaries within the alveolar walls receive deoxygenated blood from the pulmonary arteries, which is high in carbon dioxide. As the blood passes through the alveoli and reaches the pulmonary veins, oxygen is absorbed, and carbon dioxide is released, resulting in a reduced state of O_2 and CO_2. Typically, all alveoli are both ventilated and supplied with blood [2].

Heliox is a mixture of helium (He) and oxygen (O_2) that has been widely used as clinical therapy since 1934 [3]. The therapeutic benefits of heliox therapy were first studied and positively reported by Barach, who observed decreased work of breathing (WOB) in asthma patients after the heliox therapy, paving the way for current clinical uses.

Principles of Gas Exchange in the Lung

The atmosphere is composed of a mixture of gases, with s nitrogen (N_2) making up 79%, oxygen (O_2) 21%, carbon dioxide (CO_2) 0.04%, and other gases present in smaller proportions. Highly soluble gases exchange in the airways with bronchial circulation, while less soluble gases exchange in the alveoli with pulmonary blood. Solubility in water and blood affects gas exchange characteristics [4]. Ŧ

This gaseous mixture exerts a pressure known as atmospheric pressure (P_{atm}). At sea level, the total atmospheric pressure is 740 mm Hg (millimetres of mercury). It can be represented as:

$$P_{atm} = P_{N2} + P_{O2}$$

where:

Partial pressure of nitrogen (P_{N2}) = 79% × 740 mm Hg = 600 mm Hg
Partial Pressure of oxygen (P_{O2}) = 21% × 740 mm Hg = 160 mm Hg

Henry's law describes gas behaviour when it comes in contact with liquids like blood. It asserts that the amount of gas dissolved in a liquid is linked to both the gas's solubility and partial pressure. Despite nitrogen being abundant in the air, only a small amount dissolves in blood due to its low solubility in the liquid medium, as shown in Table 1 [4].

Gas exchange from the alveoli to the bloodstream happens directly through passive diffusion. This process does not involve active, transport, and no energy is required for diffusion (Figure 1). However, both ventilation and perfusion are convective process that do require energy, and in various cardiorespiratory diseases, one or both processes may be impaired [5].

Table 1. Factors influencing the solubility of major respiratory gases

Gas	Solubility (mL.dL/mm hg)
Oxygen (O_2)	0.024
Carbon dioxide (CO_2)	0.57
Carbon monoxide (CO)	0.018
Nitrogen (N_2)	0.012
Helium (He)	0.008

OXYGEN TRANSORT

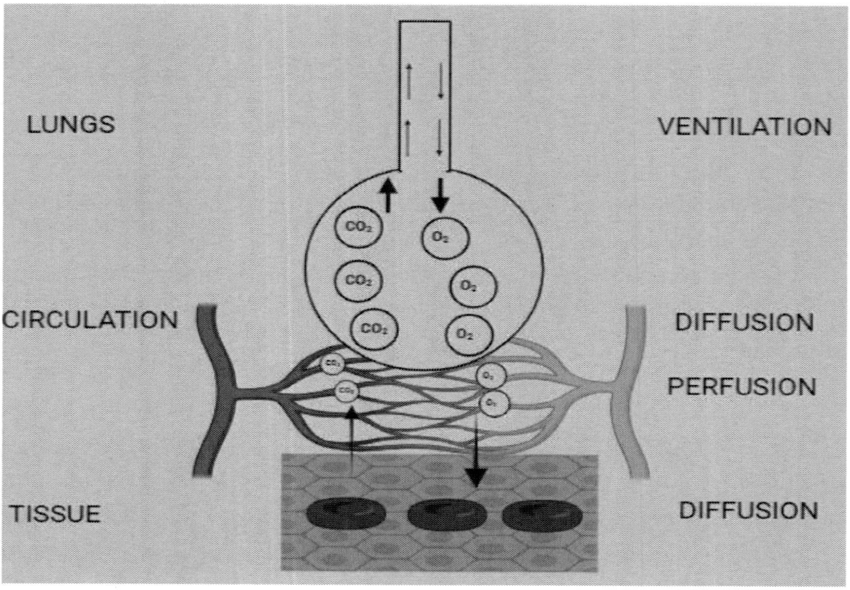

Figure 1. Diagrammatic representation of the oxygen transport process and Carbon-dioxide transport process from the tissue to the lungs. (Created by biorender.com).

Therefore, effective blood flow and ventilation in the lung are required to maintain the efficient gas exchange. Clinically, most cases of impaired gas exchange is a result from a reduced correlation between ventilation and perfusion (V_A/Q mismatch; V_A = alveolar ventilation, Q = total lung blood flow). This mismatchresults in areas of the lung being over- or under-ventilated relative to their respective blood flow rates. This chapter discuss the mechanism of gas exchange as it relates to helium therapy and how O_2 and CO_2 gas exchange efficiency is affected by V_A/Q mismatch [5].

When gas molecules are in contact with surfaces, they exert force or pressure. Gases exist in the natural environment as a mixture of several molecular types. Partial Pressure (P) refers to the pressure exerted by a single type of gas within a mixture of gases. According to Dalton's law, each type of gas in a mixture exerts its own pressure, contributing to the total pressure (P_{10}) exerted by the gas mixture, which is the sum of all partial pressures. The total pressure increases in proportion to the concentration of gas molecules overall. Understanding partial pressure is crucial for predicting gas movement. Gases naturally move from areas of higher partial pressure to areas of lower partial pressure when connected. Moreover, the greater the difference in partial pressure between two regions, faster the gases will move [6].

Mass conservation is the underlying principle that unifies the three different physical processes (1. ventilation, 2. diffusion, and 3. perfusion). This simply indicates that every oxygen molecule inhaled but not exhaled diffuses within the lung from alveolar gas to bloodstream (see Figure 1).

The product of minute ventilation (V_E, L/min) and the difference between inspired and mixed expired O_2 concentrations (FiO_2 and FeO_2, respectively) determines the volume of O_2 (VO_2) transferred from the alveolar gas to pulmonary capillary blood per minute. The amount of O_2 entering pulmonary capillaries is calculated by multiplying pulmonary blood flow (Q, L/min) by the difference between the concentration of O_2 in pulmonary venous blood ($C_{pv}O_2$) and pulmonary arterial blood (C_VO_2). This assumes homogeneity of the lungs, where the O_2 concentration in the blood leaving each alveolus remains constant, thus equating to the systematic O_2 concentration (C_aO_2).

These relationships can be expressed through simple mass conservation equation as follows:

$$VO_2 = V_E \times (FIO_2 \text{ and } FEO_2) = V_A \times (FIO_2 - FAO_2) \quad (1)$$

$$VO_2 = Q \times (C_aO2 - C_VO_2) \quad (2)$$

The right side of equation 1, establishes that the conducting airways do not participate in blood or air gas exchange. This makes it possible to substitute alveolar ventilation (VA) and alveolar O_2 concentration. We can consider the Po2 in the alveolar gas (PAO_2) and the capillary blood leaving the alveolus to be the same, since diffusion transport normally functions well within the time of red blood cells at sea level [5].

This implies that $C_{PV}O_2$ (consequently CaO_2 in the second equation) represents the oxygen concentration that can be determined directly from the HbO_2 dissociation curve at the P_AO_2 value (considering that $P_AO_2 = F_AO_2 \times k$, where k is a constant equivalent to (barometric pressure minus saturated water vapour pressure)/100).

According to Rahn and Fenn [8], the equation can be expressed using the same variable, VO_2

$$VA \times (FIO_2 - F_AO_2) = Q \times (CaO_2 - CvO_2) \quad (3)$$

If we rearrange the terms, we can express it as

$$VA/Q = 8.63 \times (CaO_2 - CvO_2) / (PIO_2 - P_AO_2) \qquad (4)$$

In this context, the constant term ensures consistency in the equation when using units such as L/min for both VA (BTPS) and Q; mL/dL (STPD) for both CaO_2 and CVO_2 and mm Hg for both PIO_2 and P_AO_2.

The discussion involves simplifying assumptions to understand gas exchange, including continuous ventilation and perfusion, lung homogeneity in VA/Q ratio, nearly identical inspired and expired gas volumes, constant oxygen concentration in blood entering the pulmonary veins, and assumed diffusion equilibration. Research suggests that their combined effect is negligible in health, but may be significant in disease states with VA and Q heterogeneity. The equations describe the relationship between alveolar and arterial gas concentrations and how changes in VA/Q ratio affect oxygen and carbon dioxide levels. Regions with low VA/Q ratios experience reduced oxygen levels, while those with high ratios have a greater effect on carbon dioxide [5].

Heliox Gas Exchange

Helium is an unreactive gas, lacks taste and odour and does not facilitate combustion or interact with biological membranes. It is the lightest gas, with density of 0.179 g/L, which is 86% less than that of room air (1.293 g/L). Helium is lighter than the nitrogen and oxygen. Hydrogen is the only gas that exhibit lower density; however, it is highly flammable. Helium's reduced density lowers the Reynolds's number associated with airflow through the airways, which signifies the correlation between the radius of the airways and the velocity, density, and viscosity of the gas. This can be expressed as

[Radius of the airway × Velocity × Density of gas] / Velocity of gas

The therapeutic benefits of utilizing helium lies in its unique physical properties, such as decreased density and heightened viscosity when compared to oxygen or nitrogen. Breathing a mixed gas of low density has many theoretical benefits for patients with breathlessness including reduced resistance to flow, improved laminar flow, and decreased pressure required to pass through airways, thereby reducing the work of breathing (WOB) [7]. Increased airway resistance can be seen in chronic obstructive pulmonary disease (COPD) due to:

1. Increased secretion in the airway (bronchia wall)
2. Inflammation of the bronchial wall
3. Reduced elasticity of the lung due to narrowing of the airways
4. These conditions lead to an increase in turbulent airflow, which occurs at low ventilation [7].

Clinically, heliox therapy has been shown to have significant therapeutic effects in the treatment of upper airway obstruction [8]. Marini [9] and Hess [10] have separately concluded in their reviews that a theoretical argument rooted in gas physics can be presented both for and against the advantage of heliox usage in conditions where the obstruction is presumed to be more peripheral. Several physical phenomena resulting from inhaling a less dense gas occur concurrently, and this, combined with differences in disease pathology between individuals, may partially explain the diverse responses documented regarding heliox. Nevertheless, heliox does not directly treat airway resistance; instead, it diminishes the amount of inspiratory pressure required by the patient or ventilator to achieve a specific gas flow. The work required to move a gas to the alveolus is reduced by one third when breathing helium gas. In general, the distinctive physical properties of helium facilitate smoother gas flow, reduced airway resistance and decreased work of breathing in patients with obstructive airflow. As an inert gas, helium does not interact with human metabolism; hence, it can be safely administered to patients without causing any adverse effects. Laude [11] conducted a study in COPD, and Ahmedzai [12] studied cancer patients by comparing a mixture of helium with oxygen and nitrogen with oxygen. They found significant improvement in oxygen saturation in both COPD and cancer patients.

Regional differences in lung diseases are expected, and areas with improved ventilation will respond more significantly to changes in gas composition. Improving overall lung ventilation and distribution could enhance oxygenation, improve ventilation/perfusion matching, and increase oxygen saturation, which could decrease ventilator requirements, respiratory rates, and reduce hyperinflation in obstructive patients [8]. A multicenter randomized trial was conducted in Canada and Europe involving ICU populations to investigate whether the use of a helium-oxygen mixture for 72 hours during non-invasive ventilation could decrease the failure rate of non-invasive ventilation requiring intubation. The trial was stopped early because helium-oxygen mixtures decreased the failure rates in both groups and improved ventilation. These improvements are likely attributed to the enhanced gas exchange facilitated by helium, which has a more favourable carbon dioxide diffusion compared to air [13].

Physical Properties of Helium

The unique physical properties of helium have significant clinical implications in respiratory diseases. Heliox is a mixture of helium and oxygen, widely used clinically to decrease airway resistance and enhance airflow rate. Helium is a common gas at room temperature and diffuses quickly due to its low atomic weight. The challenge of helium storage lies in preventing leaks due to the ineffective designs of conventional cylinders. The diffusion coefficient of helium allows carbon dioxide to diffuse more rapidly in heliox than in air or oxygen [14].

A theoretical examination conducted by Papamoschou compared flow rates of helium-oxygen mixtures (heliox) and air-oxygen mixtures. The author observed significant improvement in flow rates when helium replaced nitrogen under typical atmospheric conditions [15]. Heliox has demonstrated positive outcomes in conditions such as asthma, COPD, bronchiolitis, bronchopulmonary dysplasia, and pneumothorax [7].

The Impact of Helium Substitution in Gas Mixtures on Respiratory Physiology

Helium possesses a molar mass of 4.0 mol/L; being biologically inert, it is insoluble in human tissues at atmospheric pressure. Long-term inhalation of helium-oxygen (He-O_2) mixtures has been found to be safe, with no deleterious effects observed. Compared to nitrogen and oxygen, helium is significantly less dense being seven times less dense than nitrogen and eight times less dense than oxygen. The density of a gas mixture follows a concentration-weighted sum of its constituent parts, with density decreasing as temperature increases. Although helium, nitrogen and oxygen have roughly similar viscosities, the viscosity of gas mixtures increases with temperature. However, within the practical range of temperatures encountered in respiratory settings the differences in viscosities between nitrogen-oxygen (N_2-O^2) and He-O_2 mixtures are negligible [16].

Effects Helium on Breathing Dynamics

During spontaneous breathing, inhaled gas is warmed and humidified in the upper airway. Regardless of the method used (e.g., heated humidifier or heat-moisture exchanger), the inspired gas mixture entering the trachea approaches core body temperature with near 100% relative humidity. Water vapour, a component of expired gas, has minimal effect on the flow characteristics of gas mixtures. However, carbon dioxide in expired gas influences the Reynolds number and, hence, flow characteristics, particularly in He-O_2 mixtures with little clinical significance.

Physiological Impact of Helium Substitution

Substituting helium for nitrogen in inspired gas results in a significant decrease in the Reynolds number for mixtures with varying fractions of inspired oxygen. This leads to a higher proportion of laminar or mixed flow, resulting in increased volumes per unit time. Consequently, alveolar gas mixing is enhanced, improving collateral ventilation and alveolar unit recruitment. Moreover, the rapid diffusion of oxygen and carbon dioxide through helium compared to nitrogen leads to a more complete diffusion equilibrium, contributing to a reduction in the alveolar-arterial oxygen difference [17-18].

Effects of Helium on Gas Exchange in Healthy Individuals

During resting conditions, inhaling a helium and oxygen mixture (79:21) does not significantly alter gas exchange in normal individuals. Several studies have compared the effects of breathing heliox versus room air on healthy subjects during exertion. Although the methodologies, measurement techniques, and outcomes of these studies differ, a consistent message emerges. Esposito and Ferretti assessed respiratory parameters and gas exchange variables in eight subjects breathing four variety of gas mixtures such as air, He-O_2 (79:21), N_2-O2 (89:11) and He-O_2 (89:11) during exercise at maximum effort [16, 17].

Conclusion

Heliox therapy represents a promising approach in respiratory medicine, particularly in the treatment of conditions characterized by airway obstruction. Utilizing the unique physical properties of helium, such as reduced density and improved gas flow dynamics, heliox has demonstrated efficacy in reducing airway resistance and decreasing the work of breathing. Clinical studies have shown its potential to enhance gas exchange, improve ventilation dynamics, and contribute to better outcomes in patients with respiratory disorders. Continued research and exploration of heliox therapy holds promise for further advancements in respiratory care [18].

Key Messages

1. Heliox therapy offers potential benefits in managing respiratory conditions by reducing airway resistance and improving gas flow dynamics.
2. Gas exchange in the lungs depends on efficient ventilation and perfusion, highlighting the importance of maintaining a balance between two or optimal respiratory function.
3. The unique physical properties of helium make it an effective component of heliox therapy.
4. Clinical studies demonstrate the efficacy of heliox therapy in various respiratory conditions.
5. Understanding gas exchange principles and helium's effects informs the use of heliox therapy in respiratory care.

References

[1] Hess D. *Respiratory care: principles and practice.* Jones & Bartlett Learning; 2011 Aug 24.

[2] Wagner PD. The physiological basis of pulmonary gas exchange: implications for clinical interpretation of arterial blood gases. *European Respiratory Journal* 2015 Jan 1;45(1):227-43.

[3] Gentile MA. Inhaled medical gases: more to breathe than oxygen. *Respiratory care* 2011 Sep 1;56(9):1341-59.

[4] Wagner PD. The physiological basis of pulmonary gas exchange: implications for clinical interpretation of arterial blood gases. *European Respiratory Journal* 2015 Jan 1;45(1):227-43.

[5] Petersson J, Glenny RW. Gas exchange and ventilation–perfusion relationships in the lung. *European Respiratory Journal* 2014 Oct 1;44(4):1023-41.

[6] Esquinas AM, editor. *Pulmonary Function Measurement in Noninvasive Ventilatory Support.* Springer International Publishing; 2021 Aug 20.

[7] Valli G, Paoletti P, Savi D, Martolini D, Palange P. Clinical use of Heliox in asthma and COPD. *Monaldi archives for chest disease* 2007;67(3):159-64.

[8] Laude EA, Ahmedzai SH. Oxygen and helium gas mixtures for dyspnoea. *Current opinion in supportive and palliative care* 2007 Aug 1;1(2):91-5.

[9] Marini JJ. Heliox in chronic obstructive pulmonary disease… Time to lighten up? *Critical care medicine* 2000 Aug 1;28(8):3086-8.

[10] Hess DR. Heliox and noninvasive positive-pressure ventilation: a role for heliox in exacerbations of chronic obstructive pulmonary disease? *Respiratory care* 2006 Jun 1;51(6):640-50.

[11] Laude EA, Duffy NC, Baveystock C, Dougill B, Campbell MJ, Lawson R, Jones PW, Calverley PM. The effect of helium and oxygen on exercise performance in chronic obstructive pulmonary disease: a randomized crossover trial. *American journal of respiratory and critical care medicine* 2006 Apr 15;173(8):865-70.

[12] Ahmedzai SH, Laude E, Robertson A, Troy G, Vora V. A double-blind, randomised, controlled Phase II trial of Heliox28 gas mixture in lung cancer patients with dyspnoea on exertion. *British journal of cancer.* 2004 Jan;90(2):366-71.

[13] Kleiman AM, Huffmyer JL. Helium: Is the Sky the Limit? *Respiratory Care* 2018 Apr 1;63(4):488-90.

[14] Hess DR, Fink JB, Venkataraman ST, Kim IK, Myers TR, Tano BD. The history and physics of heliox. *Respiratory care* 2006 Jun 1;51(6):608-12.

[15] Papamoschou D. Theoretical validation of the respiratory benefits of helium-oxygen mixtures. *Respiration physiology* 1995 Jan 1;99(1):183-90.

[16] Ball JA, Rhodes A, Grounds RM. The role of helium in the treatment of acute respiratory failure. In *Yearbook of Intensive Care and Emergency Medicine 2001* (pp. 446-463). Springer Berlin Heidelberg.

[17] Erickson BK, Seaman J, Kubo K, Hiraga A, Kai M, Yamaya Y, Wagner PD. Mechanism of reduction in alveolar-arterial PO2 difference by helium breathing in the exercising horse. *Journal of Applied Physiology* 1994 Jun 1;76(6):2794-801.

[18] Erickson BK, Seaman J, Kubo K, Hiraga A, Kai M, Yamaya Y, Wagner PD. Hypoxic helium breathing does not reduce alveolar-arterial PO2 difference in the horse. *Respiration physiology* 1995 Jun 1;100(3):253-60.

Chapter 5

Heliox Basic Equipment

Mostafa Elshazly*, MD
and Eman Kamal Ibrahim, MD

Faculty of Medicine, Cairo University, Giza, Egypt

Abstract

Mixing helium and oxygen (heliox) results in a gas with lower density and a viscosity similar to that of air. Heliox converts turbulent flow to laminar flow and reduces the work of breathing, which helps decrease airway resistance and enhance ventilation. Most protocols use a helium to oxygen ratio of 70/30 or 80/20, as previous studies suggest that the high concentration of helium—usually more than 70% of the gas mixture—is necessary for heliox to effectively reduce airway resistance. There are two important technical issues that should be considered when using heliox in clinical practice or research studies. First, the differences in the density of between heliox and oxygen or air can alter the function of flow sensors of ventilators. Second, there are noteworthy changes in the delivery of nebulized drugs when using heliox as the driving gas.

There are two methods to deliver heliox in spontaneously breathing patients. The first method is an open circuit using a face mask attached to reservoir bag. The second method is a semi-closed system, which has the advantage of reducing heliox consumption and, consequently, costs. When prescribing nebulizers with heliox as the driving gas, it may result in a reduction in the size and amount of inhaled drug; therefore, the flow to nebulizer should be increased to simulate the flow of oxygen-based system.

* Corresponding Author's Email: elshazly66@hotmail.com

In: Respiratory Care in Heliox Therapy Physiology and Technology
Editor: Antonio M. Esquinas
ISBN: 979-8-89530-385-6

The use of noninvasive positive pressure ventilation (NPPV) with heliox can reduce dynamic hyperinflation and work of breathing, as well as prevent or postpone intubation and mechanical ventilation. In mechanically ventilated patients, the use of heliox can influence the flow sensors of traditional ventilators, which are designed to utilize air and oxygen, due to the low density and thermal properties of heliox. Recently, manufacturers have started introducing modifications to enable the safe delivery of heliox with new ventilators.

Keywords: heliox, airway resistant, work of breathing, aerosol delivery

Introduction

Helium was discovered in 1868 by a French astronomer Pierre Janssen, who observed a bright yellow line with a wavelength of 587.49 nm in the spectrum of the sun during a solar eclipse [1]. The element was first isolated on Earth in 1895 by a British chemist William Ramsay. Later that year, Swedish chemists determined its atomic weight [2]. Helium is a colorless, odorless, tasteless, nontoxic, inert gas with no known toxic effects even when used for extended periods. It has an atomic number of 2 and an atomic weight of 4 g/mol, allowing it to diffuse rapidly due to its low atomic weight. At room temperature, helium exists as an ordinary gas. Its low molecular weight and density allow it to pass through valves and airways with minimal turbulence. Helium's diffusion coefficient facilitates more rapid diffusion of CO_2 through heliox compared to air or oxygen.

Mixtures of helium and oxygen (heliox) were first used in diving to create breathing environments for divers at great depths, reducing the formation of nitrogen bubbles responsible for decompression illness.

Barach [3] first described the positive effects of heliox for treating patients with asthma and airway obstruction. The observation of reduced work of breathing (WOB) immediately after treatment with heliox supports its current clinical applications. After the late 1930s, little was reported about clinical applications of heliox until 1979 [4]. Since then, a variety of claims have been made regarding heliox's respiratory benefits. Heliox helps to decrease airway resistance and enhance ventilation by converting turbulent flow to laminar flow, thereby reducing the work of breathing (Figure 1).

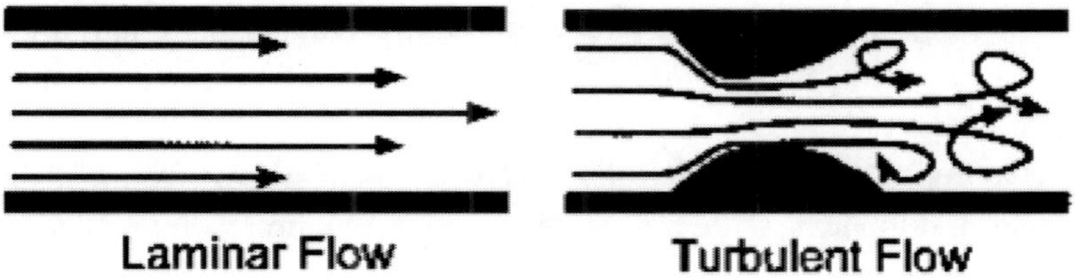

Figure 1. Graphic about turbulent flow to laminar flow.

Previous evidence suggests that the effect of heliox in reducing airway resistance requires a high concentration of helium—greater than 70% of the gas mixture [5]. Thus, the purpose of this chapter is to discuss the basic equipment for heliox delivery in different situations.

Delivery Systems

Heliox is supplied in compressed medical gas cylinders, typically available in sizes E, H, and G. Gas regulators designed specifically for helium must be used to ensure the safe and accurate delivery of heliox.

Caution is also necessary when using heliox with medical devices, as oxygen and air flow meters do not correctly measure heliox flow due to the differences in gas density. A heliox flowmeter should be utilized for delivery when available. If delivered through an oxygen flow meter, clinicians need to multiply the indicated flow by 1.8 to determine the total flow to the patient. To determine how long an H or K tank of heliox will last, therapists use the cylinder factor 2.5. The formula is:

Duration of flow (min) = Pressure (psig) X Cylinder Factor / Flow (L/min)

Heliox can be administered via nasal cannula (NC), high flow nasal cannula (HFNC), non-rebreathing mask (NRB), aerosol nebulizer, and both invasive and non-invasive mechanical ventilation.

Technical Considerations

According to Graham's law, gas flow through an orifice is inversely proportional to the square root of the gas density. Consequently, heliox flows through an oxygen flow meter at a rate 1.8 times higher than that of oxygen. Therefore, ventilators and pneumotachometers require recalibration before utilizing heliox [6].

Two important technical issues arise when using heliox in clinical practice or research studies. First, he physical properties of heliox, compared to oxygen or air, can alter the function of flow sensors on ventilators. Second, the delivery of nebulized drugs is significantly affected when using heliox as the driving gas.

The Optimal Helium-to-Oxygen Ratio

The best helium-to-oxygen ratio is not definitively known, however, most studies and treatment protocols used a mixture of helium to oxygen at 70/30 or 80/20%. In some situations, 30% oxygen may not be sufficient to correct hypoxia, and a mixture of 60/40% could be used. It is important to note that increasing the oxygen fraction may reduce the beneficial effects of heliox, making it not suitable for pulmonary diseases with high oxygen requirements, such as some parenchymal lung diseases [7].

Heliox in Spontaneously Breathing Patients

There are two ways to deliver heliox to spontaneously breathing patients. The first method is an open circuit using a face mask attached to reservoir bag, requiring an adequate flow of gas to maintain inflation (Figure 2). The disadvantages of this method include high heliox consumption— typically about 18 liters/min—to avoid re-breathing exhaled gas, contributing to the higher cost of using the open circuit [8].

The second method is a semi-closed system, which reduces heliox consumption to less than 1 liter/min, thereby reducing costs (Figure 2). However, the initial costs for equipment, nursing, and other requirements of semi-closed circuit should be considered [9].

A previous study comparing open circuit and semi-closed circuits for heliox delivery in spontaneously breathing patients revealed that the semi-closed circuit reduced costs to about one-fifth of those of the open circuit. Additional procedures required, such as aerosol therapy, nursing, nutrition and hygiene should also be factored into the overall heliox consumption w cost [10].

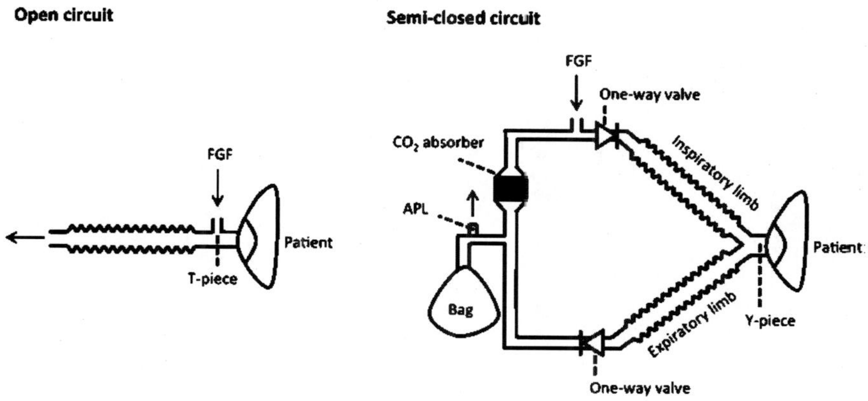

Figure 2. The illustration of an open circuit and a semi-closed circuit. FGF—Fresh Gas Flow, APL— Adjustable Pressure Limiting valve.

A disadvantage of the semi-closed system is the high gas flow, the resistance of inspiratory and expiratory limbs and the expiratory pressure limiting valve, which can increase the patient's work of breathing. To minimize system resistance, a simple water seal can be used instead of a pressure valve, but bacterial and viral filters must be removed, necessitating sterilization after each use [10].

Heliox and Aerosol Delivery

Most patients who are candidates for heliox treatment may require inhaled drugs, such as bronchodilators. Previous studies have suggested that heliox can increase the delivery of medications to the lungs, hence increasing the bronchodilator effect. However, adequate drug delivery depends on the method used for administration. Researchers recommend using nebulizers with oxygen and adding heliox as carrier gas to facilitate drug delivery. When prescribing nebulizers with heliox as the driving gas, the size and amount of inhaled drug may decrease, so the flow to nebulizer should be increased to simulate the flow of oxygen-based system [11]. Large volume heliox nebulizers are designed to be powered with oxygen while utilizating heliox as a carrier gas (Figure 3).

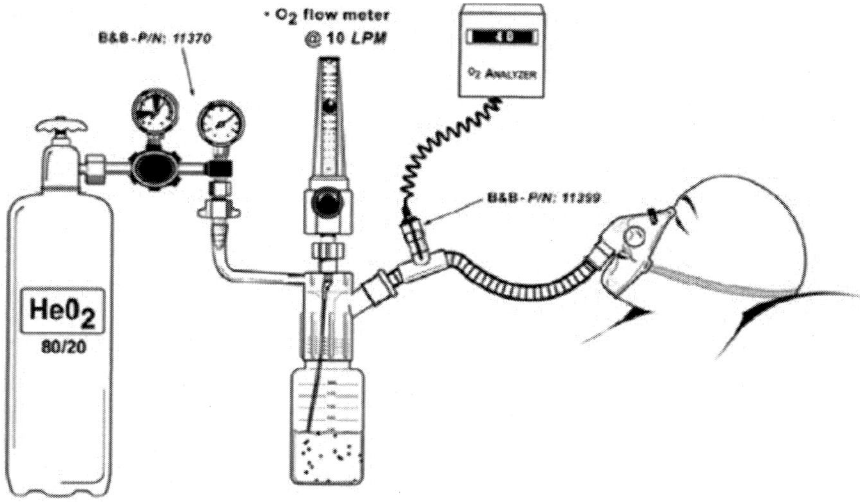

Figure 3. Large volume heliox nebulizer (B&B Medical Technologies, Loomis, California).

Heliox and Vapotherm

The Precision Flow Heliox System by vapotherm delivers heliox non-invasively through nasal cannula, providing ideal humidification and temperature to improve patient comfort and adherence. However, further studies are needed to establish the improved outcomes of heliox delivered via vapotherm in specific conditions.

Heliox and Non-Invasive Positive Pressure Ventilation (NPPV)

There is evidence that the combination of NPPV and heliox can reduce dynamic hyperinflation, work of breathing, and help prevent or postpone intubation and mechanical ventilation. The advantages of using NPPV with heliox, compared to heliox via a non-re-breathing mask, include active humidification, pressure-supported breaths, positive-end-expiratory pressure (PEEP) and continuous monitoring. Although concerns existed about the risk of malfunctioning traditional NPPV devices when using heliox, recent findings indicate that using appropriate ventilators in combination with commercially available heliox delivery systems is a safe option [12]. Single-limb circuit devices with passive exhalation should not be used due to the higher flows required, inconsistencies in the delivered fraction of inspired helium (FiHe), and the excessive cost of delivery.

Heliox and Mechanical Ventilation

To use heliox effectively with mechanical ventilation, critical issues must be addressed such as availability of technical expertise and suitable ventilators that can function adequately and safely with heliox. The use of heliox can influence the flow sensors of traditional ventilators which are designed for air and oxygen, due to heliox's low density and thermal properties. Also, tidal volumes delivered to patients may be underestimated when heliox is administrated, causing the ventilator to cycle irregularly. Gas mixing and oxygen sensors may fail to function normally during heliox delivery, resulting in continuous low oxygen and low minute volume alarms. Recently manufacturers have started introducing modifications to allow safe heliox delivery with new ventilators [13].

Heliox mechanical ventilation can be started by connecting a compressed air hose to an 80/20 heliox tank or by using a heliox blend with an oxygen concentration close to 21%. It is advisable to connect two heliox tanks so that when one is empty, they can continue to supply heliox, preventing any interruption in delivery for severely ill patients. Due to the high thermal conductivity of heliox, a heated wire circuit humidifier should be utilized, and plastic wrap around the circuit is necessary to maintain the temperature of the heliox delivered to patients. The heat wire flow sensor may malfunction with heliox use and should be disabled, complicating volume-targeted ventilation. However, the ventilator can be safely set to pressure ventilation mode, as heliox does not affect pressure measurement or delivery [14]. If a ventilator is not calibrated for heliox, its density, viscosity, and thermal conductivity may interfere with proper functioning. Caution is essential with any mechanical ventilator not calibrated for heliox, as malfuncting may occur with gases other than air and oxygen, significantly altering delivered and exhaled VT measurements [15].

A mechanical ventilator must be approved, or adequately bench-tested to ensure safe operation with heliox. It is imperative to consult the ventilator's operation manual and contact the ventilator manufacturer to guarantee the safe use of heliox.

Cost and Availability

Heliox is available in cylinders, each containing about 160 liters, with different helium-oxygen ratios of 80/20, 70/30, and 60/40. Each cylinder costs about 3.5 times the price of the same amount of oxygen or air. At a flow rate near 12-15 liters/min, non-intubated patients will require about 3- 6 cylinders per day, while mechanically ventilated patients will need about three tanks per day [8].

Conclusion

Heliox is a mixture of helium to oxygen 70/30 or 80/20% resulting in a gas with lower density and similar viscosity to air. Heliox converts turbulent flow to laminar flow and reduces the work of breathing, actions that help decrease airway resistance and enhance ventilation. When used as a driving gas during nebulization, heliox may result in a reduction in the size and amount of inhaled drug; therefore, the flow to the nebulizer should be increased to simulate the flow of an oxygen-based system. The use of NPPV with heliox can reduce dynamic hyperinflation, work of breathing, and help prevent or postpone intubation and mechanical ventilation. In mechanically ventilated patients, heliox can affect the flow sensors of traditional ventilators designed for air and oxygen due to its low density and thermal properties.

Key Messages

1. The potential therapeutic effects of heliox are related to its low density and its tendency towards laminar airflow, reducing turbulent flow airway resistance.
2. The optimal helium-to-oxygen ratio is not definitively known, although most protocols employ helium-to-oxygen ratios of 80/20 or 70/30.
3. A significant limitation of heliox is the low fractional concentration of inspired oxygen (FiO_2) in the gas mixture, which may not be suitable for patients with hypoxemia.

4. The use of heliox during mechanical ventilation requires proper calibration of the ventilator and continuous monitoring due to its distinct effects on ventilator performance.
5. There are no evidence-based guidelines regarding the use of heliox. A therapeutic trial may be acceptable in clinical conditions associated with severe airway obstruction, provisional treatment may provide a bridge to definitive treatment.

References

[1] Dean R Hess 1, James B Fink, Shekhar T Venkataraman, In K Kim, Timothy R Myers, Benoit D Tano. The History and Physics of Heliox. *Respir Care* 2006;51(6): 608–612.

[2] Emsley J. *Nature's building blocks: An A-Z guide to the elements.* New York: Oxford University Press; 2001.

[3] Barach AL. Use of heliox as a new therapeutic gas. *Proc Soc Exp Biol Med* 1934;32: 462–464.

[4] Thiriet M, Douguet D, Bonnet JC, Canonne C, Hatzfeld C. [The effect on gas mixing of a He-O2 mixture in chronic obstructive lung diseases (author's translation).] *Bull Eur Physiopathol Respir* 1979; 15(5):1053–1068.

[5] Frazier MD, Cheifetz IM. The role of heliox in paediatric respiratory disease. *Pediatric Respir Rev* 2010; 11:46–53.

[6] Oppenheim-Eden A, Cohen Y, Weissman C, Pizov R. The effect of helium on ventilator performance: study of five ventilators and a bedside Pitot tube spirometer. *Chest* 2001 Aug;120(2):582-8.

[7] Gluck EH, Onorato DJ, Castriotta R. Helium-oxygen mixtures in intubated patients with status asthmaticus and respiratory acidosis. *Chest* 1990 Sep;98(3):693-8.

[8] Roche-Campo F, Vignaux L, Galia F, Lyazidi A, Vargas F, Texereau J, Apiou-Sbirlea G, Jolliet P, Brochard L. Delivery of helium–oxygen mixture during spontaneous breathing: evaluation of three high-concentration face masks. *Intensive Care Med* 2011; 37:1787–92.

[9] Roubik K, Zazula R, Strnadova A. Spontaneous breathing of heliox using a semi-closed circuit: A bench study. *Int J Artif Organs* 2012; 35:466–70.

[10] Jurickova I, Roubík K, Muller M. Delivery of heliox with a semi-closed circuit during spontaneous breathing: a comparative economic theoretical study. *BMC Pulm Med* 2015 Jun 10; 15:65.

[11] Corcoran TE, Gamard S. Development of aerosol drug delivery with helium oxygen gas mixtures. *J Aerosol Med* 2004 Winter;17(4):299-309.

[12] Hess Dean R. Heliox and Noninvasive positive pressure ventilation: A role for heliox in Exacerbations of Chronic Obstructive Pulmonary Disease. *Respir Care* 2006;51(6):640-50.

[13] Brown MK, Willms DC. "A Laboratory Evaluation of 2 Newer Mechanical Ventilators in the Presence of Helium-Oxygen Mixtures." *Respir Care* 2005; 50(3): 354-60.

[14] Chowdhury M. M. M., Reus E., Brown M. K., Habibi P. Heliox and Ventilatory Support: What Does it Mean for the Future of Infant Care? *Infant* 2006: 2(5): 194-200.

[15] Berkenbosch, John W., Ryan E. Grueber, Osuama Dabbagh, and Andrew McKibben. Effect of Helium-Oxygen (Heliox) Gas Mixtures on the Function of Four Pediatric Ventilators. *Critical Care Medicine* 2003: 31, 2052–58.

Chapter 6

Monitoring Heliox Therapy. Basics and Rationale

Daniela Filipa dos Santos Bento*, MD
Intensive Care Medicine Department, Centro Hospitalar de Trás-os-Montes e Alto-Douro, Vila Real, Portugal

Abstract

Heliox therapy is a medical intervention that involves the administration of a mixture of helium and oxygen to patients with certain respiratory conditions. The basic rationale behind heliox therapy is rooted in the physical properties of helium and its ability to alter the flow dynamics of gases in the respiratory system. This therapy is typically considered in specific clinical scenarios where the benefits of reduced airway resistance and improved gas flow dynamics outweigh potential risks. The decision to employ heliox should be made by healthcare professionals based on a thorough assessment of the patient's clinical status and their response to other treatments. Monitoring the patient's response during therapy is crucial to ensure its effectiveness and safety. Monitoring during heliox therapy should be tailored to the specific needs of the patient and the underlying respiratory condition. Close attention to clinical signs, physiological parameters, and communication among healthcare providers is essential for optimizing the benefits of heliox therapy while minimizing potential risks.

Keywords: heliox, helium, monitoring, respiratory, airway

---

* Corresponding Author's Email: danbento@chtmad.min-saude.pt

In: Respiratory Care in Heliox Therapy Physiology and Technology
Editor: Antonio M. Esquinas
ISBN: 979-8-89530-385-6

Introduction

Heliox therapy is a medical intervention that involves the administration of a mixture of helium and oxygen to patients with certain respiratory conditions. Its first use was described by Barach in the mid-1930s - he administered helium to asthmatic patients and patients with laryngeal obstruction for relief of dyspnea [1], and since then many other applications have been studied [2]. Helium is an inert, odorless, tasteless, nontoxic, noncarcinogenic gas present in the atmosphere. The basic rationale behind heliox therapy is rooted in the physical properties of helium and its ability to alter the flow dynamics of gases in the respiratory system: lower density and viscosity enable less turbulent flow through the airways, which improves the efficiency of gas flow through narrowed orifices and decreases the work of breathing [2, 3]. Heliox does not treat airway resistance, but, rather, reduces the inspiratory pressure of the patient or ventilator required for a given gas flow. The effort required to move a volume of gas to the alveolus is reduced. Additionally, helium enhances the effect on carbon dioxide elimination, which diffuses faster with heliox than with a nitrogen/oxygen mixture. [3]. It is also used as an adjunct to traditional bronchodilator therapy. The combination of heliox and bronchodilators/ steroids can enhance the bronchodilator effects and improve overall respiratory function [3, 4].

This therapy is typically considered in specific clinical scenarios where the benefits of reduced airway resistance and improved gas flow dynamics outweigh potential risks. These scenarios may include acute exacerbations of asthma, upper airway obstruction, or other respiratory conditions with significant airflow limitation. Heliox therapy is used as a temporary intervention to provide rapid relief while other definitive treatments are initiated.

The decision to employ heliox should be made by healthcare professionals based on a thorough assessment of the patient's clinical status and response to other treatments. Monitoring the patient's response during therapy is crucial to ensure its effectiveness and safety.

Patients receiving heliox therapy should be located in a monitored unit with continuous cardiopulmonary monitoring. Clinical assessment, arterial blood gases, peak inspiratory pressure, and tidal volume (V_t) should be performed regularly [4, 5]. Benefits from the therapy are often seen quickly, usually within an hour of initiation of treatment [5, 6].

Before initiating heliox therapy, the clinical staff should have adequate training to deliver the gas and resources such as hospital policies or procedures should be on hand to guide their care. Since few institutions have heliox piped directly into the intensive care unit, most rely on cylinders of gas brought manually to the bedside. Heliox delivery equipment should be assessed by a skilled clinician at least every two hours [7].

Patient Monitoring During Therapy

We consider the following key points.

1. Continuous pulse oximetry is crucial. This helps ensure that the patient is adequately oxygenated during heliox therapy. In hypoxic patients, a balance needs to be struck between improving ventilation (by minimizing supplemental oxygen) and achieving adequate oxygenation (by diluting heliox with supplemental oxygen). Oxygenation goals should be adjusted individually.
2. Regular assessment of respiratory rate and effort should be conducted (hourly or less) [7]. Changes in these parameters can provide early indications of the patient's response; increased rate and effort may raise concern about therapy failure.
3. Assess patient comfort and tolerance. Some patients may find the heliox mixture more challenging to breathe than air, and adjustments may be necessary. Additionally, inform patients about any changes in voice pitch in non-intubated patients.
4. Check the temperature regularly. Hypothermia has been associated with the administration of heliox to infants, due to its high thermal conductivity, especially when it is administered for prolonged periods. The risk of hypothermia can be mitigated with adequate warming and humidification of the heliox, using standard devices [7].
5. Assess respiratory dynamics: An increase in tidal volume, decrease in peak inspiratory pressure, and decrease in work of breathing are indicators of therapy effectiveness. Conversely, inverse dynamics should raise suspicion about barotrauma, which can occur due to changes in gas dynamics. This assessment must consider the calibration of the device using heliox (see technical issues)
6. Perform periodic measurement of blood gases: Conduct arterial blood gas analysis periodically to assess the patient's acid-base status, oxygenation levels, and carbon dioxide levels. This helps in

determining the overall effectiveness of heliox therapy. Expected results are decrease in PaCO2 measurement with adequate PaO2.

7. Record data: Maintain detailed records of respiratory parameters, oxygen saturation levels, and any changes in the patient's clinical status. Documentation is essential for tracking progress and making informed decisions about ongoing treatment.

Technical Issues

We consider the following key points.

1. Instrument recalibration: Caution must be taken with heliox and medical devices. Oxygen and air flow meters do not correctly measure heliox flow due to the difference in gas density (the flow of gas through an orifice is inversely proportional to the square root of its density -Graham's Laws of Diffusion and Effusion). The actual flow rate of heliox through an oxygen flow meter is 1.8 times greater than the indicated flow [3, 4]. For this reason, ventilators need to be recalibrated and approved to operate with heliox. Correction factors for recalibration are available for most ventilators; however, it is imperative to consult the ventilator's operation manual or contact the ventilator manufacturer [4].
2. Titration of Heliox: The optimal helium-oxygen ratio is unknown, although most protocols recommend a mixture that includes 70 to 80 percent helium and 30 to 20 percent oxygen. Increases in the oxygen fraction tend to diminish the beneficial effect of using a low-density gas, therefore diseases with high oxygen requirements are typically not amenable to heliox [8].
3. Aerosol delivery assessment: heliox can decrease the particle size of the nebulized solution, which may enhance drug delivery to the lower airways This hypothesis has been evaluated in several studies examining lung deposition of heliox-driven aerosols in humans [9]. However, it can also negatively affect nebulizer functioning by causing insufficient flow, which results in reduced output, and longer nebulization times [8, 9]. When heliox is used in nebulization, the flow should be increased by 50–100% to ensure adequate nebulizer output [8].

4. Verify heliox availability and cost prior to start therapy: Heliox's benefits are realized only while the patient is breathing the mixture, therefore, the treatment must be continuous. Helium-oxygen mixtures come in "H" cylinders (159 cubic feet) in ratios of 80:20, 70:30, or 60:40. Each cylinder costs 3.5 times more than a similar cylinder of oxygen. Considering flow rates of 12 to 15 L/min, three to six of these cylinders may be used each day in nonintubated patients, and approximately three tanks per day in patients receiving mechanical ventilation [10]. Unexpected disruption in gas delivery can have serious consequences. When heliox is discontinued abruptly, the patient may decompensate quickly.

Other Monitoring Recommendations

We consider the following key points. Healthcare Provider Communication: Communicate regularly with the healthcare team to share information about the patient's response to heliox therapy. This collaboration ensures a comprehensive approach to patient care.

Conclusion

Monitoring during heliox therapy should be tailored to the specific needs of the patient and the underlying respiratory condition. Close attention to clinical signs, physiological parameters, and communication among healthcare providers is essential for optimizing the benefits of heliox therapy while minimizing potential risks. In summary, heliox therapy is a valuable intervention in respiratory care, and careful monitoring of clinical and physiological parameters is crucial to ensure its effectiveness and safety for patients with respiratory issues.

Key Messages

The key messages from heliox therapy monitoring can be summarized as follows:

1. Heliox therapy is primarily used in patients with acute or chronic respiratory conditions such as asthma, chronic obstructive pulmonary disease (COPD), or upper airway obstruction. The aim is to improve gas flow in the airways, reduce the work of breathing and increase the supply of oxygen to tissues.
2. Heliox is usually administered through a specialized mask or ventilation system. The concentration of helium in the mixture may vary depending on the patient's condition.
3. Regular clinical assessment is necessary to assess the patient's response to therapy: continuous monitoring of respiratory rate, heart rate and oxygen saturation and periodic analysis of blood gases help to assess the effectiveness of the therapy.
4. It is crucial to monitor for any signs of discomfort, intolerance, or adverse reactions.
5. Monitoring the resolution of symptoms of respiratory distress and improvement in overall respiratory function is an important outcome measure.

References

[1] Barach AL. The use of helium in the treatment of asthma and obstructive lesions in the larynx and trachea. *Ann Intern Med.* 1935;9:739–65.

[2] Hunt T, Williams MT, Frith P, Schembri D. Heliox, dyspnea, and exercise in COPD. *Eur Respir Rev.* 2010;19:30–8.

[3] Gentile MA. Inhaled medical gases: more to breathe than oxygen. *Respir Care.* 2011 Sep;56(9):1341-57; discussion 1357-9.

[4] Hess DR, Fink JB, Venkataraman ST, Kim IK, Myers TR, Tano BD. The history and physics of heliox. *Respir Care.* 2006 Jun;51(6):608-12.

[5] Hashemian SM, Fallahian F. The use of heliox in critical care. *Int J Crit Illn Inj Sci.* 2014 Apr;4(2):138-42.

[6] Fink JB. Opportunities and risks of using heliox in your clinical practice. *Respir Care.* 2006 Jun;51(6):651-60.

[7] Brown M, Willms D. Heliox therapy. *Yearbook Respiratory Care Clinics and Applied Technology.* 2008:153-63.

[8] Kim IK, Phrampus E, Venkataraman S, Pitetti R, Saville A, Corcoran T, et al., Helium/oxygen-driven albuterol nebulization in the treatment of children with moderate to severe asthma exacerbations: a randomized, controlled trial. *Pediatrics.* 2005;116(5):1127–33.

[9] Anderson M, Svartengren M, Bylin G, Philipson K, Camner P. Deposition in asthmatics of particles inhaled in air or in helium-oxygen. *Am Rev Respir Dis*. 1993 Mar;147(3):524-8.

[10] Hess DR, Chatmongkolchart S. Techniques to avoid intubation: noninvasive positive pressure ventilation and heliox therapy. *Int Anesthesiol Clin*. 2000 Summer;38(3):161-87.

Chapter 7

Heliox Therapy in Airway Related Problems – Resurgence of a Forgotten Gem

Dipasri Bhattacharya[1,*], MD
and Antonio M. Esquinas[2], MD, PHD, FCCP
[1]Department of Anesthesiology, Critical Care and Pain,
R. G. Kar Medical College, Kolkata, West Bengal, India
[2]Intensive Care Unit, Hospital Morales Meseguer, Murcia, Spain

Abstract

Heliox is a mixture of helium and oxygen usually used in various airway-related problems in both adult and pediatric patients with satisfactory results. Its use in obstructive airway disease shows great promise. The commercial use of helium as a carrier gas for oxygen has many advantages, such as low gas density, which significantly lowers the turbulence in gas flow in the distal parts of lung, facilitating laminar flow, and decreasing airway resistance and the work of breathing. Although it was popular in the early 1900s, the use of Heliox gradually declined in the post-World War II era, mainly due to the advancement of more potent bronchodilators. Interest in heliox resurfaced in the early 1980s when asthma-related deaths began to rise, leading to ongoing research into its broader applications in airway management, particularly for its ability to lower airway resistance. The use of heliox in conditions causing upper airway obstruction is not intended to treat the underlying pathology; but rather, it serves to reduce airway resistance and respiratory muscle workload until definitive treatment can be given. Recently, its use in managing croup in children and COVID-19-associated pneumonia has been documented.

* Corresponding Author's Email: dipasribhattacharya123@gmail.com

In: Respiratory Care in Heliox Therapy Physiology and Technology
Editor: Antonio M. Esquinas
ISBN: 979-8-89530-385-6

Keywords: heliox, airway related problems, mode of ventilation, aerosol delivery

Introduction

Helium-oxygen (Heliox) mixtures have been widely used for decades in the treatment of various respiratory disorders, ranging from acute upper airway obstructions to lower airway conditions such as asthma and exacerbations of chronic bronchitis [1]. Helium was first discovered as a bright yellow line in the sun's atmosphere by the French astronomer Janssen during a total solar eclipse. Later, the English astronomer Lockyer, observed it in the solar spectrum and named it after the Greek word for sun, "helios" [2, 3]. Helium was first isolated for commercial use from the mineral clevite in 1895 [1]. It's as a carrier gas for oxygen was first described by Barach in the early 1930s [1]. Although nitrogen and helium have comparable viscosity, helium has higher thermal conductivity. As a result, a Heliox gas mixture (79% helium and 21% oxygen) has a viscosity similar to, but a density nearly six times lower than that of atmospheric air [1]. Helium is a colorless, tasteless, non-combustible, and biologically inert gas that is insoluble in human tissues and has no bronchodilator or anti-inflammatory effects [1, 2]. It has the lowest specific gravity of any gas with the exception of hydrogen, which is highly combustible. Heliox gas mixtures are known to be non-toxic, non-carcinogenic, and have no lasting effects on human organs [1, 2, 3].

Mechanism of Action of Heliox

Gas flow in airways may be laminar, turbulent, or a combination of the two (transitional). Laminar flow is the most efficient way to deliver oxygen to the distal parts of the bronchial tree [1]. The likelihood of laminar or turbulent flow depends on the density and viscosity of the gas, expressed by the gas mixture's Reynolds number: $Re = pvr/n$ where Re is the Reynolds number, p is the density, v is the velocity, r is the cross-sectional radius, and n is the viscosity [4]. The flow type at any given point is determined by the Reynolds number. High Reynolds numbers (greater than 4000) indicate predominantly turbulent flow, while low Reynolds numbers (less than 2000) indicate principally laminar flow [4]. Within the lungs, there is a transitional region where turbulent flow becomes laminar. Heliox reduces the Reynolds number, converting turbulent flow into more efficient laminar flow, and decreases the pressure gradient needed to maintain turbulent flow, thus reducing the work of breathing [2, 3, 4]. Conditions such as exercise or any disease that increases ventilatory requirements shifts this transitional area distally, leading to greater turbulent flow [3, 4]. Due to its low density, heliox provides laminar flow, lowers resistance to gas flow within the airways and permits an increase in ventilation [4].

Adverse Effects

Due to the inert nature of helium, it does not undergo metabolism in the human body, making it safe for most patients. However, the following points must be kept in mind while using helium gas mixtures:

1. For helium to be effective, it should ideally constitute more than 70% of the inhaled gas mixture. This may limit the amount of oxygen that can be delivered, resulting in hypoxemia [1, 2].
2. Helium's high thermal conductivity may lead to a lowering of body temperature when used for prolonged periods [1, 2, 3].

Delivery Systems

Standard cylinders contain Heliox (1200 liters) in a mixture of 79% helium and 21% oxygen, which can be administered via any oxygen delivery device. However, administration is most effective via a non-rebreathing facemask, as this allows for the best concentration to be delivered to the patient without mixing with room air [1, 3, 4]. Heliox therapy for spontaneously breathing patients using a semi-closed circuit is more cost-effective compared to an open circuit [4].

Heliox and Mode of Ventilation

In controlled mechanical ventilation (CMV) and synchronized intermittent mandatory ventilation (SIMV), heliox driven volume-controlled ventilation is currently not recommended in patients requiring tidal volume (VT) <40 ml [5]. Heliox-driven pressure-controlled ventilation can be used in premature neonates with endotracheal tube (ETT) sizes of 2.0 mm internal diameter and a weight of at least 500 g. The inspired fraction of oxygen (FiO_2) should be kept to the minimum required for adequate oxygenation, in order to optimize the inspired fraction of helium (FiHe) [5]. This necessitates greater flexibility and tolerance of oxygen saturation. The aim is to achieve $FiHe \geq 0.6$, t which corresponds to $FiO_2 \leq 0.4$ when possible. If a patient is hypoxic, it is preferable to use volume recruitment strategies, such as increasing PEEP, VT, or peak inspiratory pressure (PIP) in the case of pressure-controlled ventilation before increasing FiO_2 [5, 6, 7].

The Role of Heliox in Non-Invasive Ventilation (NIV)

The use of heliox in combination with NIV in COPD patients presenting with exacerbations is a promising therapy for critically ill patients who could not be treated through other methods [7]. Helium is an inert gas with a very low density (0.18 g/L), allowing it to pass through narrowed air passages with less turbulence than nitrogen or oxygen. Heliox is extremely safe with no adverse effects [7, 8]. However, continuous monitoring is needed during heliox therapy. Heliox therapy is not a definitive treatment but rather a temporary measure until definitive treatment begins to take effect [7, 8]. Heliox administered via high flow nasal cannula (HFNC) has shown good results in the treatment of acute bronchiolitis in children [9]. Carbon dioxide elimination improves in acute respiratory distress syndrome when heliox is administered during HFNC [9].

Uses of Heliox Therapy for Airway Problems

Upper Airway Obstruction

Upper airways obstruction is the most common indication for heliox use. The literature suggests that the greater the severity of the obstruction, the greater the benefit from breathing heliox [10]. Obstruction increases airway resistance, leading to increased work of breathing, respiratory muscle fatigue, and life-threatening problems like hypercapnia and hypoxemia. Heliox facilitates laminar flow, decreasing the work of breathing [11]. Patients become less anxious, more comfortable and more cooperative as their work of breathing decreases [12].

Lower Airway Obstruction

Helium-oxygen mixtures are used to treat obstructive airway diseases in patients with croup, narrow endotracheal tubes (ETTs), respiratory distress syndrome, asthma, bronchiolitis, and acute exacerbations of chronic obstructive pulmonary disease (COPD) and acute lung injury [12, 13]. Heliox enhances gas distribution in lower airway obstructions [12, 13]. Morgan et al., [14] used heliox in 2014 to treat a case of coronavirus OC43 infection in an infant with severe acute respiratory distress, successfully avoiding intubation.

Chronic Obstructive Airway Disease

Heliox consistently improves both inspiratory and expiratory flow, reducting dynamic hyperinflation (intrinsic PEEP) and consequently improving gas exchange [15]. This reduction in hyperinflation improves mechanical advantage by increasing respiratory muscle efficiency and decreasing the work of breathing, which in turn reduces carbon dioxide production. Heliox may also enhance the bronchodilation effects of β-agonist administration for acute asthma. However, its usefulness in COPD remains under evaluation, with current evidence being inconclusive [16].

Asthma

Various studies have shown that patients with status asthmaticus unresponsive to conventional therapies may benefit from breathing heliox until definitive therapies take effect. TWhile many studies favor heliox as an emergency intervention for alleviating breathing difficulty in asthma, there are also conflicting results [16].

Croup (Acute Laryngotracheobronchitis)

Croup is an age specific viral infection of the upper and lower respiratory tracts, causing inflammation in the subglottic area, which results in dyspnea and stridor. Studies by Weber et al., [17] and Moraa et al., [18] have demonstrated the beneficial effect of heliox in children with croup, especially those who are refractory to racemic epinephrine, showing reductions in croup scores and improvements in respiratory distress [17, 18].

Vocal Cord Dysfunction

Heliox reduces airway resistance and may result in rapid improvement in patients with acute vocal cord dysfunction [19, 20]. Its relatively low cost and minimal adverse effects make heliox an appropriate choice [20].

Subglottic Stenosis

Heliox can prevent intubation in subglottic stenosis by initiating laminar flow through the rigid tube and reducing the work of breathing [21].

Difficult Intubation

With a lower density than air or oxygen, heliox improves airflow through constricted passages. The effective heliox concentration should ideally be >60%, with gas flows meeting or exceeding the inspiratory flow demands of the patient to avoid dilution with room air [22]. Intrinsic endotracheal or endobronchial disease can lead to significant airway difficulties due to obstruction and loss of available lung for oxygenation and ventilation. In cases of a large anterior mediastinal mass, heliox aids in preoxygenation of the patient by initiating laminar flow [22]. In congenital diaphragmatic hernia, heliox improves oxygenation when used in conjunction with mechanical ventilation [23].

Use in Tracheostomy

Heliox administered via laryngeal mask airway (LMA) can be used for tracheostomy under conscious sedation in extremely anxious patients [24]. The use of heliox during tracheostomy has been documented in podiatric patients with severe upper airway obstruction [25].

COVID-19 Infection

Heliox therapy has demonstrated a high degree of reliability in improving blood oxygenation and normalization of the acid-base balance, thereby enhancing efficacy and reducing treatment time in COVID-19 associated pneumonia [26, 27].

Aerosol Delivery

Currently available nebulizers are designed to operate with nitrogen-oxygen mixtures. Using heliox may affect the nebulizer's performance by decreasing the density of the gas mixture. It has been reported that powering a nebulizer with heliox decreases the fraction of the total dose and the respirable mass of the drug compared to using air. In a pediatric model of mechanical ventilation, a 70:30 heliox mixture provided better deposition of albuterol from a metered dose inhaler (MDI) than oxygen-enriched air, [28, 29].

Nonconventional Ventilation

Heliox has been found to be beneficial in various forms of nonconventional ventilation, including high-frequency oscillatory ventilation (HFOV), high-frequency jet ventilation, and high-frequency percussive ventilation [30].

Conclusion

Despite more than 60 years since Barach first described the use of helium-oxygen mixtures for managing obstructive disorders of the respiratory tract, its use remains sporadic and undefined. However, there is significant interest and potential for application in combination with new respiratory therapies, such as nasal high-flow oxygen, non-invasive mechanical ventilation and in specific clinical subgroups with upper airway disorders, serving as a "bridge" to support gas exchange and work of breathing in severe, acute and chronic respiratory disorders.

Key Messages

1. The physical properties of helium make it an ideal carrier gas for oxygen in place of nitrogen for various respiratory conditions.
2. The low density and viscosity of heliox promote smoother gas flow, reduce airway resistance, and decrease the work of breathing in selected patients.
3. There is evidence supporting its use alongside conventional treatments in asthma, COPD, croup, and other respiratory conditions, although further research is needed to define its precise role. Heliox is cost-effective due to low gas consumption and can be combined with all ventilator modes, including controlled mechanical ventilation, non-invasive ventilation, and high flow nasal oxygen therapy.

References

[1] Reuben AD, Harris AR. Heliox for asthma in the emergency department: a review of the literature. *Emerg Med J* 2004; 21:131–135.
[2] Rodrigo G, Rodrigo C, Pollack C, Travers A.. Helium-oxygen mixtures for nonintubated acute asthma patients. *Cochrane Library*. Issue 4. Oxford: Update Software, 2001.
[3] W. M. Haynes, ed., *CRC Handbook of Chemistry and Physics*, CRC Press/Taylor and Francis, Boca Raton, FL, 95th Edition, Internet Version 2015, accessed December 2014.
[4] Ball JAS, Rhodes A, Grounds RM. A review of the use of helium in the treatment of acute respiratory failure. *Clinical Intensive Care* 2001; 12:105–13.
[5] Chowdhury MM, Brown MK, Habibi P. Heliox and ventilatory support: What does it mean for the future of infant care? *Infant* 2006; 2:194–203.

[6] Berkenbosch JW, Grueber RE, Dabbagh O, McKibben AW. Effect of helium oxygen (heliox) gas mixtures on the function of four pediatric ventilators. *Crit Care Med* 2003; 31:2052–8.

[7] Hurford WE, Cheifetz IM. Respiratory controversies in the critical care setting. Should heliox be used for mechanically ventilated patients? *Respir Care* 2007; 52:582–91.

[8] Dani C, Fontanelli G, Lori I, Favelli F, Poggi C. Heliox non-invasive ventilation for preventing extubation failure in preterm infants. *J Matern Fetal Neonatal Med* 2013; 26:603–7.

[9] Seliem W, Sultan AM. Heliox delivered by high flow nasal cannula improves oxygenation in infants with respiratory syncytial virus acute bronchiolitis. *J Pediatr (Rio J)* 2018 Jan-Feb;94(1):56-61.

[10] Chan PK, To KF, Wu A, Tse GM, Chan KF, Lui SF, Sung JJ, Tam JS, Tomlinson B. Human metapneumovirus-associated atypical pneumonia and SARS. *Emerg Infect Dis* 2003;10(3):497-500.

[11] Truebel H, Wuester S, Boehme P, Doll H, Schmiedl S, Szymanski J, Langer T, Ostermann T, Cysarz D, Thuermann P. A proof-of-concept trial of HELIOX with different fractions of helium in a human study modelling upper airway obstruction. *European Journal of Applied Physiology* 2019; 119:1253–1260.

[12] McGarvey JM, Pollack CV. Heliox in airway management. *Emerg Med Clin North Am* 2008; 26:905–20.

[13] Beurskens CJ, Wösten-van Asperen RM, Preckel B, Juffermans NP. The potential of heliox as a therapy for acute respiratory distress syndrome in adults and children: a descriptive review. *Respiration* 2015; 89:166-174.

[14] Morgan S, Vukin K, Mosakawoski S, Solano P, Stanton L, Lester L, Lavani R, Hall JB and Tung A. Use of Heliox Delivered via High-Flow Nasal Cannula to Treat an Infant with Coronavirsu- Related Respiratory Infection and Severe Acute Air-flow Obstruction. *Respir Care* 2014;59 (11):e166-1170.

[15] Weder A, Gaspar S, Chiappa R. Heliox improves minute-ventilation variability during incremental maximal exercise in COPD patients. *Manual Therapy Posturology & Rehabilitation Journal* 2023; 21.1255.

[16] Mutlu GM, Budinger GR. Not much turbulence: Addition of heliox to noninvasive ventilation fails to improve outcomes in patients with exacerbations of chronic obstructive pulmonary disease. *Crit Care Med* 2010;38:319–20.

[17] Weber JE, Chudnofsky CR, Younger JG, Larkin GL, Boczar M, Wilkerson MD, Zuriekat GY, Nolan B, Eicke DM. A randomized comparison of helium-oxygen mixture (Heliox) and racemic epinephrine for the treatment of moderate to severe croup. *Pediatrics* 2001;107:E96.

[18] Moraa I, Sturman N, McGuire TM, van Driel ML. Heliox for croup in children. *Cochrane Database Syst Rev* 2021 August16;8(8):CD006822.

[19] Balkissoon R, Kenn K. Asthma: Vocal cord dysfunction (VCD) and other dysfunctional breathing disorders. *Semin Respir Crit Care Med* 2012; 33:595–605.

[20] Deckert J, Deckert L. Vocal cord dysfunction. *Am Fam Physician* 2010; 81:156–9.

[21] Connolly KM, McGuirt WF., Jr Avoiding intubation in the injured subglottis: The role of heliox therapy. *Ann Otol Rhinol Laryngol* 2001; 110:713–7.

[22] Galway U, Doyle DJ, Gildea T. Anesthesia for endoscopic palliative management of a patient with a large anterior mediastinal mass. *J Clin Anesth* 2009; 21:150–1.

[23] Wise, A. C., Boutin, M. A., Knodel, E. M., Proudfoot, J. A., Lane, B. P., Evans, M. L., Suttner, D. M., & Kimball, A. L. Heliox adjunct therapy for neonates with congenital diaphragmatic hernia. *Respiratory Care* 2018; 63(9): 1147–1153.

[24] Daumerie G, Stacey Su, Ochroch EA. Anesthesia for the Patient with Tracheal Stenosis. *Anesthesiology Clin* 2010;28: 157–174.

[25] Okkeş Ozgür Mar, Dincer Yildizdas, Ozden Ozgur Horoz, Faruk Ekinc. Use of Heliox therapy in a child with tracheostomy who developed respiratory distress due to bronchiolitis associated with respiratory syncytial virus. *Cukurova Medical Journal* 2020;45(3):1257-0.

[26] Manuilov VM, Suvorov AV, Kurkin SV, Olenev YO, Pavlov NV, Logunov AT Anikeev DA, Orlov OI. Evaluation of the Efficiency of Oxygen-Helium Therapy for Patients with Covid-19-Associated Pneumonia. *Hum Physiol* 2022;48(7):863-870.

[27] Wang, T., Xiang, Q., & Bian, J. Promising gas therapies for severe COVID-19. *Journal of Intensive Medicine* 2021; 1(2): 1–4.

[28] Bigham MT, Jacobs BR, Monaco MA, Brilli RJ, Wells D, Conway EM, Pettinichi S, Wheeler DS. Helium/oxygen-driven albuterol nebulization in the management of children with status asthmaticus: A randomized, placebo-controlled trial. *Pediatr Crit Care Med* 2010; 11:356–61.

[29] Dailey PA, Harwood R, Walsh K, Fink JB, ThayerT, Gagnon G, & Ari A. Aerosol delivery through adult high flow nasal cannula with heliox and oxygen. *Respiratory Care* 2017; 62(9): 1186–1192.

[30] Gupta VK, Grayck EN, Cheifetz IM. Heliox administration during high- frequency jet ventilation augments carbon dioxide clearance. *Respir Care* 2004; 49(9):1038–1044.

Chapter 8

Aerosol Therapy Using Heliox

Mohamad F. El-khatib*, PhD, MB, RRT
Department of Anesthesiology and Pain Medicine, American University of Beirut, School of Medicine and Medical Center, Beirut, Lebanon

Abstract

Traditionally, bronchodilators have been nebulized with air or oxygen. In recent years, heliox-driven bronchodilator nebulization has gained wider use in clinical practice. Due to its physical characteristics, heliox has the potential benefit of carrying aerosols deeper than air or oxygen into the distal airways during severe airway obstruction which might translate to higher deposition at the medication site of action in the distal lung and, therefore, greater bronchodilation effect at a relatively fast time. However, heliox-driven bronchodilator nebulization therapy continues to have some disadvantages and limitations.

Keywords: heliox, nebulization, aerosol therapy, lung diseases

Introduction

Heliox is a gas mixture composed of helium and oxygen. The most common heliox concentration is an 80:20 blend (79% helium: 21% oxygen). Helium is an inert, nontoxic gas that is lower in density than nitrogen and oxygen. Heliox has a low viscosity which makes it easier to breathe in comparison to atmospheric air. Heliox has been used to reduce the impact of airway

* Corresponding Author's Email: mk05@aub.edu.lb

In: Respiratory Care in Heliox Therapy Physiology and Technology
Editor: Antonio M. Esquinas
ISBN: 979-8-89530-385-6

resistance, to improve respiratory mechanics, and to decrease the work of breathing and energy expenditures in patients with a wide range of obstructive lung diseases [1]. An interesting role of heliox in the treatment of obstructive lung diseases is as a vehicle for the administration of inhaled bronchodilators and corticosteroids. This chapter will discuss the role and benefits of heliox in aerosol therapy, its indications, its administration methods, and potential limitations.

Role and Benefits of Heliox in Aerosol Therapy

Delivery of inhaled bronchodilators to more compromised distal airways via conventional methods is difficult because airway obstruction causes preferential delivery to central, less affected airways. Because of its low viscosity and less resulting turbulence, Heliox can promote a more uniform delivery and deposition of medications in the central and peripheral airways, improving delivery to the most affected areas that limit airflow. Heliox-driven delivery of bronchodilators can be particularly useful in acute asthma and COPD exacerbations [2, 3]. When compared with oxygen for delivery of inhaled bronchodilators, heliox resulted in enhanced improvement in all spirometry parameters and particular improvements in FEV1 as well as in inspiratory capacity [2]. Heliox-driven can be superior to air-driven bronchodilator therapy particularly in asthmatic patients with baseline $FEV_1 \leq 50\%$ in whom heliox-driven bronchodilator therapy induced significant increases in FVC, FEV1, FEV1/FVC, FEF25–75%, FEFmax, FEF25%, FEF50%, and FEF75% from their baseline values [4].

The lower density of heliox allows higher flow through obstructed airways at a given pressure gradient, in either turbulent or near-turbulent flows. This should allow better ventilation of and aerosol delivery to the smaller airways and alveoli particularly in patients with obstructive lung diseases like asthma and COPD [5]. Also, the lower density of heliox prevents the transition from laminar to turbulent flow. A laminar flow would have less resistance in the lung and may result in increased aerosolized medication delivery to and deposition in the lung periphery [5].

Heliox affects the delivery of medications that are administered via either nebulization or a metered dose inhaler. With heliox-driven nebulization of bronchodilators, the time for complete nebulization is prolonged, the particle size of nebulized medications is decreased, and deposition of medications is increased. For a given flow rate, the use of heliox as a driving gas instead of compressed air for nebulizing medications results in a lower pressure drop across the nebulizer orifice. This is the main reason for lower inhaled mass of medication or longer nebulization time to deliver the same amount of drug [6]. As such it is recommended that when heliox is used as a driving gas for nebulization, the flow rate should be increased by approximately 50 percent [6, 7]. However, heliox can decrease the particle size of the nebulized bronchodilator, which may enhance drug delivery to the lower airways. When used in stable asthma patients or patients with induced bronchoconstriction, heliox-driven nebulized therapy resulted in significantly lower oral deposition as well as higher particle retention in the lungs at 24 hours [8, 9]. In a small study involving 32 subjects with stable moderate-to-severe asthma, the deposition of radiolabeled bronchodilators to the middle and lower lung fields was not significantly different between heliox- or oxygen-driven nebulized therapy and enhanced deposition was observed only when positive expiratory pressure was used [2]. However, a more recent larger study including 132 patients indicated that improvements in pulmonary function test variables are more frequent and profound with heliox-driven compared to air-driven bronchodilator therapy only in asthmatic patients with baseline $FEV_1 \leq 50\%$ [4].

Indications for Heliox in Aerosol Therapy

The use of heliox for aerosol therapy may be considered in the following conditions:

a) *Acute Severe Asthma*: Heliox can be used as an adjunctive therapy to standard treatment in patients with acute severe asthma exacerbations, especially when there is poor response to initial bronchodilator therapy [10].
b) *COPD exacerbations*: In patients with severe COPD exacerbations and significant airway obstruction, heliox may help improve gas flow and decrease the work of breathing [11].
c) *Upper Airway Obstructions*: Heliox can be beneficial in cases of upper airway obstruction, such as croup or post-extubation stridor, by facilitating improved airflow and reducing respiratory distress [12].
d) *Other Obstructive Lung Diseases*: Heliox may be considered in other obstructive lung diseases such as bronchiolitis or cystic fibrosis, where airway resistance is increased [13].

Administration Methods

Heliox can be administered in various ways, depending on the patient's condition and the desired therapeutic effect. It is preferred that a heliox flowmeter is utilized for the delivery of heliox. If delivered through an oxygen flow meter, the clinician will need to multiply the flow indicated by 1.8 to determine the total flow of heliox to the patient.

a) Nebulized medications: Aerosolized medications, such as bronchodilators or corticosteroids, can be mixed with heliox and delivered through a nebulizer. The heliox gas mixture helps optimize drug delivery and depositions in the lower airways [1, 5].
b) Continuous positive airway pressure (CPAP) or Bi-Level Positive Airway Pressure (BiPAP): Heliox can be used in conjunction with CPAP or BiPAP devices to improve gas flow and decrease work of breathing in patients with respiratory insufficiency [7].
c) High Flow Nasal Cannula (HFNC): Heliox can be combined with HFNC therapy to enhance oxygenation and reduce the work of breathing [14].

Limitations and Considerations

Heliox usually comes in "H" cylinders (159 cubic feet) in ratios of 80:20 or 70:30. Its use in clinical practices can be affected by several limitations and considerations that healthcare workers should be aware of.

1. Cost: Heliox can be more expensive than standard medical gases, which may limit its use in some healthcare settings.
2. Availability: Heliox may not be readily available in all healthcare facilities, especially in resource-limited settings.
3. Monitoring: Close monitoring of the patient's clinical response, including oxygenation, respiratory rate and work of breathing, is essential when using heliox, as individual patients' responses may vary.
4. Safety: Heliox should be used with caution in patients with known helium or oxygen sensitivities or in those who are at risk of gas trapping, such as patients with bullous lung disease or pneumothorax.

Conclusion

Heliox plays a beneficial role in aerosol therapy by improving gas flow, enhancing aerosol delivery and deposition, and decreasing the work of breathing in various respiratory conditions. It can be used as an adjunctive therapy in acute severe asthma, COPD exacerbations, upper airway obstruction, and other obstructive lung diseases. However, its use should be guided by healthcare professionals and tailored to the individual patient's needs.

Key Messages

1. Heliox may provide some advantages in delivering nebulized bronchodilators in patients with obstructive lung diseases.
2. Successful heliox-driven aerosol therapy depends on several factors such as the appropriate patient selection, disease severity, and methods of administration.

References

[1] Kleiman, A. M., & Huffmyer, J. L. Helium: Is the Sky the Limit? *Respiratory Care* 2018, 63(4), 488–490.

[2] Alcoforado L, Brandaõ S, Rattes C, Brandaõ D, Lima V, et al., Evaluation of lung function and deposition of aerosolized bronchodilators carried by heliox associated with positive expiratory pressure in stable asthmatics: a randomized clinical trial. *Respir Med* 2013;107(8):1178-1185.

[3] Kress JP, Noth I, Gehlbach BK, Barman N, Pohlman AS, Miller A, et al., The utility of albuterol nebulized with heliox during acute asthma exacerbations. *Am J Respir Crit Care Med* 2002;165(9): 1317-1321.

[4] El-Khatib MF, Jamaleddine G, Kanj N, Zeineddine S, Chami H, Bou-Akl I, Husari A, Alawieh M, Bou-Khalil P. Effect of heliox- and air-driven nebulized bronchodilator therapy on lung function in patients with asthma. *Lung* 2014;192(3):377-83.

[5] Corcoran TE, Gamard S. Development of aerosol drug delivery with helium oxygen gas mixtures. *J Aerosol Med* 2004;17(4):299–309.

[6] Hess DR, Acosta FL, Ritz RH, Kacmarek RM, Camargo Jr CA. The effect of heliox on nebulizer function using a beta-agonist bronchodilator. *Chest* 1999;115(1):184-9.

[7] Hess D, Chatmongkolchart S. Techniques to avoid intubation: noninvasive positive pressure ventilation and heliox therapy. *Int Anesthesiol Clin* 2000;38(3):161-87.

[8] Anderson M, Svartengren M, Bylin G, Philipson K, Camner P. Deposition in asthmatics of particles inhaled in air or in helium-oxygen. *Am Rev Respir Dis* 1993;147(3):524-8.

[9] Svartengren M, Anderson M, Philipson K, Camner P. Human lung deposition of particles suspended in air or in helium/oxygen mixture. *Exp Lung Res* 1989;15(4):575-85.

[10] Rodrigo GJ, Castro-Rodriguez JA. Heliox-driven β2-agonists nebulization for children and adults with acute asthma: a systematic review with meta-analysis. *Ann Allergy Asthma Immunol* 2014;112(1):29-34.

[11] Gerbeaux P, Gainnier M, Boussuges A, Rakotonirina J, Nelh P, Torro D, Arnal JM, Jean P. Use of heliox in patients with severe exacerbation of chronic obstructive pulmonary disease. *Crit Care Med* 2001;29(12):2322-4.

[12] Diehl JL, Peigne V, Guérot E, Faisy C, Lecourt L, Mercat A. Helium in the adult critical care setting. *Ann Intensive Care* 2011;1(1):24.

[13] van Haren EH, Lammers JW, Festen J, van Herwaarden CL. Bronchodilator response in adult patients with cystic fibrosis: effects on large and small airways. *European Respiratory Journal* 1991 4: 301-307.

[14] Seliem W, Sultan AM. Heliox delivered by high flow nasal cannula improves oxygenation in infants with respiratory syncytial virus acute bronchiolitis. *J Pediatr (Rio J)* 2018;94(1):56-61.

Chapter 9

Heliox Therapy in Upper Airway Disorders

Doo Woong Choi[1], MD
Kevin G. Lazo[2,*], DO
and Antonio M. Esquinas[3], MD
[1]Department of Medicine, Englewood Hospital, Englewood, NJ, USA
[2]Division of Pulmonary Medicine, Englewood Health Physician Network, Bergen Medical Alliance, Englewood, NJ, USA
[3]Intensive Care Unit, Hospital Morales Meseguer Molina Segura, Murcia, Spain

Abstract

The upper airway consists of the mouth, nose, pharynx, larynx. It involves various functions including phonation, swallowing, and tasting. Obstructive events in the upper airway can lead to respiratory distress causing asphyxia and demise of the patient. The use of Heliox was 1st reported in the 1930s as a rescue therapy, and as a potential bridge to definitive treatment for upper airway obstructions in the critical care setting. This chapter will provide a brief overview of applications of Heliox therapy in upper airway disorders.

Keywords: heliox, helium, upper airway disorders

* Corresponding Author's Email: Kevin.Lazo@ehmchealth.org

In: Respiratory Care in Heliox Therapy Physiology and Technology
Editor: Antonio M. Esquinas
ISBN: 979-8-89530-385-6

Introduction

The upper respiratory airway consists of the nose, nasal cavity, and the pharynx. The pharynx is further subdivided into the nasopharynx, oropharynx, and laryngopharynx.

The nose is composed of an external portion and an internal portion which is housed inside the skull. It is made of bone as well as a series of cartilages and divided in half by the nasal septum. Generally, the nasal septum is straight at birth, however, as the patient ages, it is possible for the septum to deviate onto one side either iatrogenically or via trauma. This may cause obstruction of the nasal cavity making breathing difficult. The nasal cavity comprises three folds of tissues: the superior, middle, and inferior nasal conchae. The conchae greatly increase the surface area of the mucous membranes over which air travels.

The pharynx is a concave muscular passage connecting the oral and nasal cavities and the head to the larynx and the esophagus and the neck. The nasopharynx portion extends from the choanae in the nasal cavity down to the soft palate. The posterior nasopharynx also houses the tonsils, which are lymphoid tissues that can hypertrophy and cause airflow obstruction. The oropharynx extends from the soft palate to the epiglottis. It serves as the main channel for passage of food to the esophagus and the flow of air to the larynx. The laryngopharynx portion extends from the epiglottis to the esophagus and passes posterior to the larynx.

Dysfunctions of the musculature of the pharynx can cause speech aberrations, airflow obstructions, regurgitation of gastric contents through the nose/mouth, and aspiration into the lower airways.

Upper Airway Dysfunction Signs and Symptoms

Upper and lower airway obstructions may similarly present with shortness of breath, noisy breathing, wheezing, and diminished breath sounds. However, for upper airway obstructions, patients may be asymptomatic for a prolonged period of time, or it can present acutely. Acute presentations of upper airway obstruction may result in asphyxia and death within minutes to hours [1].

Dyspnea and noisy breathing are the most common room symptoms of upper airway obstruction and typically present during exercise, or they manifest during changes in body position such as while lying supine (e.g., sleep disordered breathing). In the latter instance there may be signs and symptoms of daytime somnolence, bilateral lower extremity edema, chronic hypoxia and hypercarbia.

Table 1. Causes of upper airway obstruction[1]

Infection – Deep Cervical Space Infections – Epiglottis – Laryngotracheobronchitis (Croup) and Bacterial Tracheitis – Tuberculosis
Upper Airway Tumors – Head and Neck Cancers – Tracheal Cancers
Laryngeal and Tracheal Stenosis – Postintubation and Posttracheotomy Stenosis (PITS and PTTS) – Post Extubation Stridor – Granulomatosis with Polyangitis - Subglottic Stenosis – Sarcoidosis - Granulomatous infiltration of the upper airways – Amyloid pseudotumor – Relapsing Polychondritis – Tracheopathia osteopathica – Idiopathic laryngotracheal stenosis
Tracheomalacia
Extrinsic Compression of Central Airway – Mediastinal masses and lymphadenopathy – Neck and Thyroid Related Causes – Diseases of the Esophagus – Vascular Abnormalities
Foreign Body Aspiration
Trauma – Facial injuries – Laryngotracheal injuries – Endotracheal Tube related injury
Inhalational Injuries
Neuromuscular disorders
Bilateral vocal cord paralysis
Vocal Cord Dysfunction
Angioedema

The normal transverse internal diameter of the trachea ranges between 15 and 25 mm in males and 10 to 21 mm in females. Clinically significant upper airway obstructions may present when the airway diameter at the site of obstruction is likely to be reduced to about 8 mm [1]. Dyspnea at rest often develops (along with stridor) when the airway diameter is about 5 mm. Stridor is a loud, musical sound of constant pitch that usually indicates the presence of extra thoracic airway obstruction most often affecting the larynx or upper trachea.

Causes of upper airway obstruction are listed in Table 1 [1].

Heliox in Upper Airway Disorders

Heliox is a mixture of 79% Helium and 21% oxygen. It is inexpensive and has minimal side effects, which makes it possible to be utilized in a variety of clinical settings. The rationale for the use of Heliox in upper airway disorders is to promote a reduction in the work of breathing for the patient. Heliox is a mixture of helium and oxygen which results in a lower density gas than pure oxygen [2]. By using a lower density gas mixture, inspiration of this gas will result in a conversion of predominantly turbulent flow at the site of upper airway obstruction to a more laminar pattern. Laminar flow would require a smaller pressure gradient than turbulent flow to achieve the same flow rate which would therefore decrease the amount of work of breathing. For example, one of the earliest uses of helium as a therapeutic gas was published in 1935 in the *Annals of Internal Medicine* [3]. There, the author administered Heliox to asthmatic patients with laryngeal obstruction for the relief of dyspnea [3].

The goal of Heliox thus, is meant to be more of a "bridge" to therapy until something more definitive can be performed to address the underlying etiology of the upper airway obstruction. Helium in an 80:20 ratio with oxygen (Heliox) was reported to be given for conscious sedation and awake intubation by Milner at al. in 1997 via a laryngeal mask airway in a patient with Gardner syndrome who had severe tracheal obstruction requiring an urgent tracheostomy [4].

Many other case reports and clinical trials have reported use of Heliox in a variety of clinical settings. One descriptive study used Heliox in the critical care setting for over 4 years in academic center in both adult and pediatric populations [5]. The study divided the data into upper airway and lower airway ailments. Heliox was used for upper airway obstruction in 43 patients, which included 16 adult patients and 27 pediatric patients. When divided by conditions, among them included nine post-extubation stridor cases, three laryngotracheobronchitis cases, two static encephalopathy cases, one tracheomalacia case, one obstructive sleep apnea case, and two non-specific stridor cases. The mean duration of Heliox use was 2.9 +/- 2.3 hours. Caregivers continued Heliox therapy for the following reasons: decreasing work of breathing (24 patients), improving hypercarbia (eight patients), improving oxygenation (15 patients), decreasing respiratory rate (18 patients), and decreasing stridor (three patients).

Regarding evidence for symptom improvement, a double-blinded randomized controlled trial was performed on pediatric trauma and burn ICU patients in post-intubation. Patients, less than 15 years old, electively extubated, with post-extubation stridor, but requiring less than 35% oxygen were studied. The study population included 13 children with 15 extubations. Stridor scores were lower with helium-oxygen compared to oxygen supplementation only (2.8 vs 3.7, $p < 0.005$). This study showed a lower stridor score with Heliox use and with no adverse effects [6].

To our knowledge no clinical trials have been performed on the use of heliox for fixed upper airway obstructions due to endotracheal/mediastinal masses. These clinical scenarios are associated with fixed upper airway obstructions that places the patient at high risk for airway compression. One case report showed successful application of heliox to a pediatric patient (two-year old girl) with a mediastinal mass that was successfully weaned from mechanical ventilation using 70:30 heliox [7].

One of the most extensively studied and common uses of Heliox is for Croup in children. A 2021 Cochrane review looked at three randomized controlled trials featuring 91 children over the duration of seven to 16 months, all studied in ER departments using 70:30 Heliox. One study showed no difference in mean respiratory rate and heart rate after 20 minutes of 70:30 Heliox for mild croup in 15 children after 20 minutes of therapy; however, all children were discharged. In another study, 47 children with moderate croup received one dose of oral dexamethasone (0.3 mg/kg) with either heliox for 60 minutes or no treatment. Heliox improved croup scores and respiratory rate 60 minutes but not at 120 minutes. In the third study, 29 children with moderate to severe croup all received continuous cool mist and intramuscular dexamethasone (0.6 mg/kg). They were then randomized to receive Heliox 70:30 + saline nebulized versus 100% FiO2 oxygen supplementation + nebulized adrenaline - gas therapies were administered for three hours each. Heliox may slightly improve croup scores at 90 minutes post intervention but may result in little or no difference overall [8].

Key Messages

1. Heliox has been utilized in a variety of upper airway obstruction cases as demonstrated by multiple case series and small randomized controlled trials.
2. Application of Heliox was reported in patients with Post-extubation stridor, Laryngotracheobronchitis, static encephalopathy, tracheomalacia, obstructive sleep apnea, non-specific stridor cases.
3. One randomized controlled trial demonstrated the role of Heliox in post-intubation symptom improvement in pediatric trauma and burn unit.
4. Three randomized controlled trials performed for children with Croup, showing heliox may slightly improve croup scores at 90 minutes post intervention, but may result in little or no difference overall.
5. The best use for Heliox may not be as a primary therapy but as a bridge to more definitive treatments for upper airway obstruction.

Conclusion

Many other case reports of Heliox can be found in the literature. Heliox may continue to have a use for a variety of upper airway obstructions, but its best use may not be as a primary therapy but as a bridge to more definitive treatments for upper airway obstruction.

References

[1] Dibiasi E, Won C, Kryger M. Chapter 47 Upper airway obstruction in adults. *Fishman's Pulmonary Diseases and Disorders*, 6 ed.

[2] Hunt T, Williams MT, Frith P, Schembri D. Heliox, dyspnoea and exercise in COPD. *Eur Respir Rev* 2010;19:30–8.

[3] Barach AL. The use of helium in the treatment of asthma and obstructive lesions in the larynx and trachea. *Ann Intern Med* 1935;9:739–65.

[4] Milner QJ, Abdy S, Allen JG. Management of severe tracheal obstruction with helium/oxygen and a laryngeal mask airway. *Anaesthesia* 1997 Nov;52(11):1087-9.

[5] Berkenbosch JW, Grueber RE, Graff GR, Tobias JD. Patterns of helium-oxygen (heliox) usage in the critical care environment. *J Intensive Care Med* 2004;19(6): 335-344.

[6] Kemper KJ, Ritz RH, Benson MS, Bishop MS. Helium-oxygen mixture in the treatment of postextubation stridor in pediatric trauma patients. *Crit Care Med* 1991;19(3):356-359.

[7] Bigham MT, Nowak JE, Wheeler DS. Therapeutic application of helium-oxygen and mechanical ventilation in a child with acute myelogenous leukemia and airway obstruction. *Pediatr Emerg Care* 2009;25(7):469-472.

[8] Moraa I, Sturman N, McGuire TM, van Driel ML. Heliox for croup in children. *Cochrane Database Syst Rev* 2021; Aug 16;8(8):CD006822.

Chapter 10

Heliox Therapy in Acute Exacerbation of Obstructive Pulmonary Disorders

Alejandro Úbeda Iglesias*, MD, PhD
and Álvaro Alonso Iglesias, MD
Department of Critical Care, Punta de Europa University Hospital, Algeciras, Spain

Abstract

Obstructive pulmonary disease involves different disorders such as chronic obstructive pulmonary disease (COPD), asthma, and bronchiolitis, all characterized by the obstruction of airflow. Based on the above, it seems reasonable to consider heliox therapy (helium and oxygen), whose physical properties allow the conversion of turbulent flow into laminar flow, thereby achieving better airflow in the distal airway. Different systematic reviews have been conducted to study this, but the results are disparate, primarily based on small-group trials or the difficulty in demonstrating different outcomes. Heliox plays an important role in patients with severe COPD in various settings, such as rehabilitation and exercise outside the hospital or in acute exacerbations requiring admission to the hospital or intensive care unit, related to the use of non-invasive ventilation. Acute bronchiolitis and heliox are also being studied, with different results. Heliox has clear benefits in the first minutes of this pathology, but these benefits have not been demonstrated in the late phase of it. In conclusion, heliox and obstructive pulmonary disease need more studies with more patients and consistent outcomes to be a real routine option in the management of these pathologies, although selected patients could benefit from its use.

---

* Corresponding Author's Email: alubeda@gmail.com

In: Respiratory Care in Heliox Therapy Physiology and Technology
Editor: Antonio M. Esquinas
ISBN: 979-8-89530-385-6

Keywords: COPD, obstructive pulmonary disorders, heliox, bronchiolitis, rehabilitation

Introduction and Definitions

Obstructive pulmonary disorders encompass a group of respiratory conditions characterized by the partial or complete obstruction of the airways, leading to difficulties in breathing and airflow limitation.

These disorders, which include asthma, chronic obstructive pulmonary disease (COPD), and bronchiectasis, pose significant challenges to respiratory function and overall well-being. Understanding the underlying mechanisms, diagnostic approaches, and effective management strategies for obstructive pulmonary disorders is crucial for healthcare professionals to provide comprehensive care and improve the quality of life for individuals affected by these conditions.

Asthma, a chronic respiratory condition, stands as a significant health challenge globally, impacting millions of individuals across all age groups. Characterized by inflammation and constriction of the airways, asthma manifests with recurring episodes of breathlessness, wheezing, coughing, and chest tightness. The next chapter will specifically address this pathology, focusing on its pathophysiology and the use of heliox as an adjunctive therapy.

COPD is a prevalent and debilitating respiratory condition that significantly impacts the lives of millions worldwide. Characterized by persistent airflow limitation and inflammation of the airways, COPD encompasses chronic bronchitis and emphysema.

Currently, COPD is an increasingly important cause of morbidity, disability, and mortality worldwide. Adeloye et al., conducted a systematic review with the aim of understanding the prevalence; it was observed that the global prevalence of COPD among people aged 30-79 years in 2019 was 10.3% (95% CI 8.2-12.8) using the GOLD (Global Initiative for Chronic Obstructive Lung Disease) case definition, which translates to 391 million people (95% CI 312.6-487.9), and 7.6% (5.8-10.1) using the LLN (Lower Limit of Normality) definition, which translates to 292 million [1].

It is significant to note about this disease, whose prevalence increases with age, presumably secondary to exposure over time to different agents, leading to its development and being more common in men [2].

Bronchiectasis, a chronic respiratory condition, unfolds as a persistent and often progressive dilation of the bronchi, resulting in impaired clearance of mucus and recurrent respiratory infections.

Bronchiolitis, a common respiratory illness predominantly affecting infants and young children, presents as inflammation and congestion of the small airways in the lungs, known as bronchioles. Giving rise to inflammation and obstruction within these delicate air passages.

Heliox is a specialized gas mixture of helium and oxygen, and it has emerged as a noteworthy component in the realm of respiratory therapy. This application is based on the physical properties of one of its components, helium.

Helium, an inert and lighter-than-air gas, holds intriguing properties that extend beyond its popular use in balloons. Comprising a mere 0.0005% of Earth's atmosphere, helium is a relatively scarce element. The main characteristics are its low density and non-reactive nature, which make it unique. Notably, the discovery of helium dates back to the late 19th century, specifically in 1868 for a French astronomer during a study of a total solar eclipse, and its journey into medical applications began in the early 20th century by Barach in 1930, who used the heliox mixture for the treatment of upper airway obstruction. Its safety profile and its beneficial effects on respiratory physiology made its use fashionable in the past for the treatment of various airway obstructions, although over time, its use has fallen out of favor due to the lack of clear evidence for improving different therapeutic endpoints identified in various clinical trials [3].

Pathophysiology Foundations

The pathophysiology of obstructive diseases encompasses a complex array of processes that affect the airways and compromise pulmonary function, from airway narrowing to chronic inflammation.

The narrowing of the airway implicates a change in the type of airflow in these, resulting in turbulent airflow at this level, which hinders the passage of air and consequently complicates the diffusion of various gases essential for basal gas exchange. In this situation, helium, as a lower-density gas, has less resistance to flow and can exhibit a laminar flow with an improvement in the narrowing airway, and can help transport various medications during acute moments to the more distal airways. It's fundamental to this physical property to talk about the Reynold number, which determines the transition from laminar flow to turbulent flow (Figure 1) [4].

As it can be observed, with a lower gas density, the Reynolds number will be smaller. Therefore, knowing that a Reynolds number < 2000 predicts laminar flow, while a Reynolds number > 3000 predicts turbulent flow, assuming that the remaining variables in the equation are constant when comparing two gases, Helium can play a fundamental role in this process, achieving laminar flow in areas of greater constriction based on its low density.

$$Re = \frac{2Vrp}{\eta}$$

Figure 1. Reynolds number. V= velocity, r=radius, p=density, μ= viscosity.

Obstructive Pulmonary Disorders and Heliox

COPD is a high-prevalence disease, and according to the World Health Organization (WHO), COPD is the third leading cause of death worldwide, causing 3.23 million deaths in 2019. Unfortunately, it is expected to be the leading cause of death worldwide by 2030. Therefore, the effective management of COPD exacerbations is crucial to improving the quality of life and reducing the burden of the disease [5].

In patients with moderate-to-severe acute exacerbations of COPD, non-invasive ventilation (NIV) is routinely used. Currently, different studies and trials, especially in children, are trying to demonstrate the benefit of heliox combination with NIV, which can even be considered synergistic. As a positive pressure, NIV can help reduce the load on respiratory muscles, prevent or correct atelectasis, prevent airway collapse, and promote and facilitate the distribution of heliox throughout obstructed airways.

Helium-oxygen can further reduce the work of breathing and improve CO_2 elimination. It can also provide higher expiratory flow than air-oxygen mixtures at the same pressure, which, in turn, can help improve passive expiratory lung mechanics, reducing the risk of barotrauma by gas trapping and thereby limiting any deleterious side effects from CPAP in obstructed airways. Application of continuous positive pressure can lower the patient's FIO_2 requirements, enabling them to be treated with a higher concentration of helium and, consequently, increasing the likelihood of treatment success. The reduction in the oxygen requirements further protects the lungs.

Jolliet et al., [6] conducted an open trial in 16 intensive care units in patients with COPD exacerbation and use of NIV, concluding that heliox improves respiratory acidosis, encephalopathy, and the respiratory rate more quickly than air/O_2 but does not prevent NIV failure. Overall, the rate of NIV failure was low.

The main problem in day-to-day practice is that the use of NIV and heliox requires specific equipment in accordance with various guidelines, ensuring proper functionality. All of this entails an increase in costs and thus poses a challenge for its routine use, and heliox must be administered with vigilance and continuous monitoring to avoid technical complications.

Furthermore, NIV with heliox theoretically embodies a new strategy for lung treatment and protection, and studies exploring this possibility should be warranted [7].

If NIV is insufficient, some patients may require intubation and connection to mechanical ventilation (IMV). In this case, heliox also plays a role, as demonstrated in various studies, by increasing airflow in areas of higher resistance. Consequently, it has been shown to reduce PEEP and respiratory effort, as well as decrease intrathoracic pressure and airway resistance, thereby improving hemodynamics and facilitating the withdrawal of invasive mechanical ventilation.

Short-term use of heliox in combination with NIV in a small study in patients with exacerbations of COPD showed benefits on work of breathing and gas exchange, but larger controlled studies of the use of heliox at COPD exacerbations are required [8].

Other studies have demonstrated a decrease in hospital stays and costs, although they require a larger number of included patients.

Lee et al., [9] conducted a study including 10 patients with pulmonary arterial catheters and severe COPD and acute respiratory failure with persistent intrinsic positive end-expiratory pressure (PEEPi) induced hemodynamic changes despite ventilator management; heliox decreased mean pulmonary arterial pressure, right atrial pressure and pulmonary arterial occlusion pressure, and increased cardiac index.

Leatherman et al., [10] enrolled 13 patients with autoPeep > 8, and they found that heliox had no effect on the degree of dynamic hyperinflation of mechanically ventilated subjects with severe air-flow obstruction. Its data suggested that heliox was unlikely to offer a clinically meaningful benefit for patients with COPD who required mechanical ventilation.

Another benefit of heliox is its use as a carrier for various medications, especially bronchodilators, in the lower airway. A study performed to compare the bronchodilator effects of albuterol and ipratropium bromide through nebulization showed that the use of heliox as a driving gas for the updraft nebulization of bronchodilators during the first 2 hours of treatment of an acute COPD exacerbation failed to improve FEV1 faster than the use of compressed room air. The faster improvement in FEF25-75 during the first 2 hours of treatment was small and of uncertain clinical significance. Despite this, heliox has demonstrated its benefit as a carrier in other pathologies, especially in asthma. Therefore, it is likely that studies with a larger number of patients will be required to establish these benefits in COPD [11].

Patients with COPD experience a complex extubation, prolonging the time under mechanical ventilation and consequently increasing the morbidity and mortality among them. Considerable literature exists describing modalities that assist in weaning COPD patients from invasive ventilation. In various studies, heliox has been used to aid in respiratory weaning with an early extubation to NIV. Heliox use has also been shown to decrease re-intubation in at least two studies.

The use of heliox outside the hospital also plays a fundamental role. Several groups of investigators have reported that the use of heliox in patients with moderate or severe COPD is associated with improved exercise performance. These improvements are primarily attributable to reductions in end-expiratory lung volume or dynamic hyperinflation, which contributes to the increased work of breathing in COPD patients. Furthermore, the resulting reduced intrathoracic pressure improves hemodynamic and peripheral oxygen delivery.

These studies have shown varied benefits of heliox on dyspnea and dynamic hyperinflation. The novel aspect of the study by Laude and colleagues [12] was the objective of evaluating the short-term effects of the contribution of each gas to dyspnea and exercise capacity.

Patients with COPD were tested in a crossover manner with heliox 28 (72% He/28% O2), heliox 21 (79% He/21% O2), 28% oxygen, or air. The main results showed that endurance walking distance improved by 64% when inspired heliox 28, compared with Heliox 21 or 28% oxygen, and all these three treatments showed improvements in exercise capacity compared with exercising on air alone [8].

Further interaction analysis showed that the beneficial effect of increasing the inspired oxygen concentration was independent of the response when using the heliox mixtures. An interesting finding of this study is that with heliox 28 the walking distance showed a skewed distribution, indicating that patients with the most severe COPD had the greatest improvements in exercise capacity [8, 11].

The most promising use of heliox mixtures would be as an adjunct to pulmonary rehabilitation in patients with severe COPD, who are still disabled by dyspnea and are unable to achieve the full benefits of training, despite pharmacologic treatment and ambulatory oxygen therapy. It could be an effective non-pharmacological tool to enhance the efficacy of rehabilitation programs, since its administration to COPD patients usually enhances their exercise tolerance, at least at a constant work rate, and thus can be useful to increase the level of physical training. The conflicting results that have been obtained so far suggest that further research is needed in order to identify the COPD patients who may be able to benefit from this kind of rehabilitation program.

Hunt et al., [13] conducted a systematic review and explored whether symptom modification and exercise performance in COPD were modified by inhalation of heliox. They summarized those eight studies that supported the effectiveness of heliox in improving the intensity and endurance of exercise.

Further studies are also needed to verify the utility of heliox as an ergogenic aid to training in pulmonary rehabilitation [8].

Acute Bronchiolitis and Heliox

In bronchiolitis, there is mixed respiratory failure, with an obstructive component due to edema and inflammation of the small airway, causing increased resistance to airflow, and a restrictive component with decreased lung compliance. The administration of heliox can be beneficial as it contributes to reducing airway resistance throughout the airway, thus decreasing respiratory work. Additionally, by facilitating carbon dioxide diffusion, it may contribute to an improvement in ventilation [4].

In 2015, Cochrane published a systematic review on the use of heliox in acute bronchiolitis. Seven randomized studies comparing heliox treatment to air oxygen in patients with bronchiolitis were reviewed (six in the pediatric-ICU and one in the emergency department). A total of 447 children under 2 years of age with acute respiratory failure secondary to bronchiolitis were included. Patients treated with heliox showed clinical improvement in the respiratory difficulty score in the first hour after the start of treatment, regardless of the mode of administration [4].

Four studies used the clinical asthma score modified by Wood: Cambonie 2006, Hollmann 1998, Kim 2011, and Martinón Torres 2008, totaling 138 patients. They demonstrated a decrease in the score of -1.04, 95% CI -1.6 to 0.48, $p = 0.0003$. However, the sample heterogeneity in these studies was high, especially due to differences in patients' baseline scores and the use of different versions of the Wood-modified score. It is noteworthy that only two studies ensured inter-observer agreement on the clinical respiratory difficulty score. No reduction in intubation rate, hospital admissions, or duration of stay in the pediatric-ICU or the duration of treatment for respiratory difficulty was found (although a reduction in the duration of treatment for respiratory difficulty was observed in a subgroup of patients who required CPAP from the beginning due to severe respiratory difficulty). No adverse effects from the administration of heliox were observed in any study [4].

The available evidence suggests that the administration of heliox may be useful alongside conventional treatment in acute bronchiolitis. This benefit is observed in the reduction of the clinical respiratory difficulty score only in the first hour of treatment, and no benefits are confirmed in gas exchange, in the need for mechanical ventilation (invasive or non-invasive), or the duration of stay in the pediatric ICU. The significant reduction in the duration of treatment for respiratory difficulty in patients with severe bronchiolitis requiring NIV from the beginning, it seems promising, suggesting that heliox may be useful when administered in NIV to the most severe patients.

More studies are needed to carefully select indications. These studies should be conducted in patients under 12 months of age with at least moderate respiratory difficulty, defined by an objective score by at least two observers.

Kuitunen et al., [14] conducted a systematic review and meta-analysis published in January 2022 and concluded that it was not justified to continue using heliox to treat bronchiolitis outside RCTs to avoid escalation of care or to shorten the hospital stay. It is possible that some patients with low respiratory capacity might benefit from the reduced breathing work, although the initiation of heliox should never delay intubation when required. It must be noted that one study found that heliox was only beneficial if it was given with a tight-fitted face mask instead of a nasal cannula. In conclusion, they found low-quality evidence that heliox does not reduce the need for NIV, intubation, or length of hospitalization in infant bronchiolitis. Although heliox seems to have short-term effects on relieving respiratory distress symptoms rapidly after its initiation, it does not have a positive effect on clinically relevant outcomes compared to standard treatment with an air-oxygen mixture.

A well-designed RCT in patients with severe bronchiolitis and proper, tight-fitting face mask administration is needed to assess whether heliox would reduce the need for NIV or endotracheal intubation.

Unlike in other pathologies, such as asthma, the use of heliox as a carrier for bronchodilators has been demonstrated not to be an effective therapy in patients with acute bronchiolitis.

In intubated patients with bronchiolitis, Kneyber et al., [15] published findings in 2009 on 13 infants ventilated with Heliox under sedation and pressure ventilation. A decrease in resistance from 69.1 ± 6.9 cm H_2O/L/sec to 50.2 ± 6 cm H_2O/L/sec ($p = 0.02$) was observed 30 minutes after starting Heliox. Static compliance and peak expiratory flow did not change.

Conclusion

Heliox plays a promising role in COPD and its exacerbations, but it can also assist patients with significant limitations in their daily lives. This could lead to an improvement in the morbidity associated with COPD, which may be crucial in managing the overall mortality linked to this condition. Heliox has also demonstrated an improvement in the first few minutes of its application in various direct and indirect parameters related to the obstruction that occurs during acute bronchiolitis.

However, the results beyond that are not consistent, and therefore, studies with a larger number of patients are necessary to assess the benefit of heliox in these pathologies.

Key Messages

1. Heliox, based on its reliable physical and physiological theories, supports the assertion that helium can improve ventilator function, especially by reducing the resistance of the airways, which is considered the main physiopathology element of obstructive syndromes.
2. Nevertheless, currently, the level of evidence does not permit a formal recommendation to be made regarding the use of heliox in the different obstructive pulmonary disorders. Despite this, heliox may

have a significant role in rehabilitation of COPD and the improvement of the exercise in severe COPD.

3. Numerous questions may be answered, in the future, concerning the use of heliox. For instance, which patients may benefit from its use? Is helium efficient in the long term in combination with NIV, IMV, or with aerosol delivery?
4. No heliox administration device should be used clinically without ample training and bench testing. One of the main limitations of heliox therapy is its accessibility and the need for specific equipment, which makes its routine use impractical in most hospital departments.
5. Heliox use seems to require more research based on clinical practice and observation through vaster investigations.

References

[1] Adeloye D, Song P, Zhu Y, Campbell H, Sheikh A, Rudan I; NIHR RESPIRE Global Respiratory Health Unit. Global, regional, and national prevalence of, and risk factors for, chronic obstructive pulmonary disease (COPD) in 2019: a systematic review and modelling analysis. *Lancet Respir Med* 2022; 10:447-58.

[2] GBD Chronic Respiratory Disease Collaborators. Prevalence and attributable health burden of chronic respiratory diseases, 1990-2017: a systematic analysis for the Global Burden of Disease Study 2017. *Lancet Respir Med* 2020;8:585-96.

[3] Arias OJ, Salas FJ, Salas-Segura DA. Uso del heliox en las crisis asmáticas moderadas y severas en el Servicio de Emergencias del Hospital Rafael Ángel Calderón Guardia. Un estudio prospectivo. *Neumol Cir Torax* 2012;71:21-8.

[4] Llorente, AM. Heliox, ¿un gas terapeútico?. *Rev Esp Ped* 2017 ;73(supl.1):54-8.

[5] Khan KS, Jawaid S, Memon UA, Perera T, Khan U, Farwa UE, Jindal U, Afzal MS, Razzaq W, Abdin ZU, Khawaja UA. Management of Chronic Obstructive Pulmonary Disease (COPD) Exacerbations in Hospitalized Patients From Admission to Discharge: A Comprehensive Review of Therapeutic Interventions. *Cureus* 2023;15:e43694.

[6] Jolliet P, Ouanes-Besbes L, Abroug F, Ben Khelil J, Besbes M, Garnero A, et al., A Multicenter Randomized Trial Assessing the Efficacy of Helium/Oxygen in Severe Exacerbations of Chronic Obstructive Pulmonary Disease. *Am J Respir Crit Care Med* 2017;19:871-80.

[7] Martinón-Torres F. Noninvasive ventilation with helium-oxygen in children. *J Crit Care* 2012;27:220.e1-9.

[8] Hashemian SM, Fallahian F. The use of heliox in critical care. *Int J Crit Illn Inj Sci* 2014;4:138-42.

[9] Lee DL, Lee H, Chang HW, Chang AY, Lin SL, Huang YC. Heliox improves hemodynamics in mechanically ventilated patients with chronic obstructive

pulmonary disease with systolic pressure variations. *Crit Care Med* 2005;33:963–73.

[10] Leatherman JW, Romero RS, Shapiro RS. Lack of Benefit of Heliox During Mechanical Ventilation of Subjects with Severe Air-Flow Obstruction. *Respir Care* 2018;63:375-9.

[11] Wedzicha JA. Heliox in chronic obstructive pulmonary disease: lightening the airflow. *Am J Respir Crit Care Med* 2006;173:825-6.

[12] Laude EA, Duffy NC, Baveystock C, Dougill B, Campbell MJ, Lawson R, Jones PW, Calverley PM. The effect of helium and oxygen on exercise performance in chronic obstructive pulmonary disease: a randomized crossover trial. *Am J Respir Crit Care Med* 2006;173:865-70.

[13] Hunt T, Williams MT, Frith P, Schembri D. Heliox, dyspnoea and exercise in COPD. *Eur Respir Rev* 2010;19:30-8.

[14] Kuitunen I, Kiviranta P, Sankilampi U, Salmi H, Renko M. Helium-oxygen in bronchiolitis-A systematic review and meta-analysis. *Pediatr Pulmonol* 2022;57:1380-91.

[15] Kneyber MCJ, van Heerde M, Twisk JWR, Plotz FB, Markhors DG. Heliox reduces respiratory system resistance in respiratory syncytial virus induced respiratory failure. *Crit Care* 2009;13:R71.

Chapter 11

Asthma Exacerbation and Heliox Therapy

Alejandro Úbeda Iglesias*, **MD, PhD**
and Álvaro Alonso Iglesias, MD
Department of Critical Care, Punta de Europa University Hospital, Algeciras, Spain

Abstract

Helium is the second most abundant element in the universe, playing an important role in the field of medicine. A mixture of helium and oxygen, known as heliox, is used for patients with various airway obstructions, particularly those with asthma, who experience turbulent flow in the smaller airways, representing a high-resistance state. During turbulent flow, lower-density gases exhibit less resistance to flow. It is estimated that approximately 339 million people worldwide suffer from asthma, making it one of the most common chronic diseases in childhood. Different studies have been conducted and published regarding heliox and its use in asthma, especially as an adjuvant therapy. However, these studies have yielded varied results, and most don't recommend heliox due to the non-significant differences observed in various outcomes. Currently, routine use of heliox is not recommended according to the guidelines for the acute management of asthma in emergency services. However, for patients who do not respond to treatment during a severe asthma attack, heliox may be considered as an adjunctive therapy, especially to improve the delivery of conventional inhaled therapies to the distal airways.

Keywords: asthma, heliox, critical asthma, heliox-driven, adjunctive therapy

---

* Corresponding Author's Email: alubeda@gmail.com

In: Respiratory Care in Heliox Therapy Physiology and Technology
Editor: Antonio M. Esquinas
ISBN: 979-8-89530-385-6

Introduction

Helium is the second most abundant element in the universe, following hydrogen. Its discovery dates back to the observation of spectral lines in the sun in 1868 by the French astronomer Jules Janssen and, independently, by British astronomer Sir Norman Lockyer. However, its isolation on Earth did not occur until 1895, when chemists Sir William Ramsay and Lord Rayleigh conducted experiments revealing its presence in radioactive minerals. Helium is relatively rare on Earth, representing 0.000524% of the atmosphere [1]. It's a colorless, odorless, inert gas, and the second lightest element in the universe. In its gaseous state, helium is exceptionally light and has a low boiling point, making it an ideal medium for a variety of medical applications.

Helium's low density allows sound waves to travel faster through it than through air, a property utilized in medical imaging technologies. Beyond its scientific curiosity, helium plays a crucial role in medicine, where it leverages its unique physical properties to advance therapeutic and diagnostic procedures.

Heliox in Medicine

Mixtures of helium and oxygen (heliox) were first physiologically used to create breathing environments for divers, reducing the formation of nitrogen bubbles responsible for decompression illness (the bends) in deep-sea divers. In the early 1930s, Barach pioneered the use of heliox the treating adults and children with asthma and upper airway obstruction. However, it was not until the 1980s that heliox regained popularity, likely due to rising mortality from asthma. The situation led to an increase in clinical trials studying heliox in different scenarios involving airway obstruction [2].

The specific concentrations of heliox used in medical settings can vary depending on the patient's clinical condition and the severity of airway obstruction. Common heliox mixtures typically range from 20% to 80% oxygen, with the remainder being helium. Greater severity of airway obstruction requires a higher concentration of helium (e.g., 80/20 for severe obstruction versus 60/40 for mild obstruction).

Heliox can be administered via a nasal cannula, a high flow nasal cannula, a non-rebreathing mask, or invasive and non-invasive mechanical ventilation. Clinicians should inform patients and their families that the patient's speech may sound squeaky during the use of heliox due to the faster sound wave speed of helium, but will return to normal after the gas is removed. If available, a helium analyzer should be used for monitoring gas delivery, but it should be recalibrated to air and oxygen routinely [3].

Several ventilator models have heliox capability, delivering and measuring heliox blends accurately. Heliox can be adapted to any ventilator by connecting the high-pressure air hose to the heliox tank. During heliox ventilation, lower driving pressures are needed to distribute oxygen to the distal alveoli for improved oxygenation and increased carbon dioxide diffusing capacity. Close monitoring is essential due to helium's significant effect on the fraction of inspired oxygen (FiO_2) delivery, displayed inspiratory tidal volume (VT), pressures, and delivered VT during both volume- and pressure-controlled ventilation. If available, use of a helium mode on the ventilator is recommended [3].

The success of heliox therapy depends on the methods and devices used. Risks of inadequate heliox administration include hypothermia (temperature <36°C for long periods), anoxia (FiO_2 lower than 21%), and delivering high lung volume, since heliox flows faster than air or oxygen, leading flow meters designed for the latter to give incorrect readings [4].

Heliox is particularly advantageous in cases of airway obstruction or respiratory distress, as its lower density reduces airway resistance, facilitating easier breathing, especially in conditions such as asthma, chronic obstructive pulmonary disease (COPD), and other respiratory disorders.

Pathophysiological Issues in Asthma

Asthma is a chronic respiratory condition characterized by airway inflammation and constriction, leading to recurrent episodes of wheezing, breathlessness, chest tightness, and coughing. It affects people of all ages, with a global prevalence on the rise. According to the World Health Organization (WHO), approximately 339 million people worldwide suffer from asthma. Although asthma mortality decreased by 59% between 1990 and 2015, the decline is not significant in certain groups, such as women over 65. Asthma is one of the most common chronic diseases in childhood, with higher prevalence rates in industrialized and urbanized countries. Significant differences also exist between countries and communities within the same region, influenced by factors such as allergen exposure, air pollution, genetics, and other environmental conditions [5].

The pathophysiology of asthma involves complex inflammatory and bronchoconstrictive processes. Airway inflammation is characterized by immune cell infiltration, inflammatory mediator release, and activation of immune responses. Airway hyperresponsiveness leads to bronchoconstriction, where the smooth muscles surrounding the airways excessively contract, narrowing the bronchial tubes.

Airway remodeling, characterized by thickening of the airway walls, increased mucus production, and alterations in the cellular composition, contributes to the chronic nature of asthma and may result in persistent airflow obstruction. The mainstays of acute asthma therapy are inhaled β-2 agonists and systemic steroids, and this combination is often sufficient alleviate acute episodes. The β-2 agonist is the primary acute treatment and causes an immediate reduction in small airway resistance through bronchial smooth-muscle relaxation and the resultant bronchodilatation. Corticosteroids have 2 different mechanisms of action. In the first few hours after administration, glucocorticoids cause upregulation of β-2 receptors on bronchial smooth muscle cells, allowing for increased efficacy of β-2 agonist therapy to reduce bronchoconstriction. Following this early effect, the anti-inflammatory effects of glucocorticoids lead to a decrease in inflammatory cytokines and reduce airway swelling [5].

Unfortunately, some patients continue to experience severe bronchospasm and respiratory distress despite initial treatment with β-2 agonists and steroids. Status asthmaticus and acute severe asthma are common terms used to describe severe or life-threatening exacerbations where bronchospasm and respiratory distress persist. Status asthmaticus occurs in approximately 20% of pediatric asthma hospitalizations. Expert guidelines from the National Institutes of Health (NIH) recommend additional adjunct therapies, for patients failing to improve with standard treatments [5].

Heliox and Asthma

Heliox is a logical option in the treatment of acute exacerbations of asthma, given the disease's pathophysiology and helium's physical properties. In asthmatics, turbulent flow in smaller airways creates a high-resistance state. During turbulent flow, lower-density gases encounter less resistance. The transition from laminar to turbulent flow is determined by the Reynolds number, based on the airway diameter, viscosity, and density. Gases with a lower density are more likely to exhibit laminar flow, particularly in large diameter airways or with higher viscosity.

Heliox is a low-cost gas mixture whose specific activity is a function of its exchange for nitrogen (approximately 79% of atmospheric air) in the respiratory system. Helium, being 7 times lighter than nitrogen, results in less dense gas (with a nominal viscosity change), improving flow during turbulent states and facilitating low-resistance laminar flow through small airways. The effect of heliox therapy should be rapid, as nitrogen is washed out of the airways within a few breaths. Once laminar flow is achieved, maximal benefit has been achieved. Since oxygen has a similar weight to nitrogen, the benefits of heliox decrease as oxygen concentration in the airway increases, reducing gas exchange efficiency.

Various studies have explored heliox's use in asthma as an adjuvant therapy, with mixed results. Most trials focus on pediatric populations due to asthma's higher prevalence in children. While heliox plays an important role in severe asthma crises, current guidelines do not recommend routine heliox therapy routinely for asthma excerbations, and its use has declined in recent years [6].

A 1996 randomized trial [7] demonstrated no significant clinical outcome differences with heliox (70% helium/30% oxygen) in hospitalized pediatric asthma subjects, although there was a small improvement in peak expiratory flow. Another randomized trial showed that heliox (80% helium/20% oxygen) improved dyspnea scores. In a study of intubated asthmatics, the addition of heliox to the ventilator circuit significantly decreased both peak inspiratory pressures and $PaCO_2$. In 2018, Leatherman et al., [8] reported that heliox administration resulted in a reduced $PaCO_2$ and peak inspiratory pressures without affecting hyperinflation indices (plateau pressure and total PEEP).

Conversely, a 2003 Cochrane review of six studies (five adult or mixed ages and one pediatric) found no significant differences in pulmonary function for subjects receiving heliox in emergency departments. A subsequent 2010 trial involving 42 children admitted to the pediatric ICU found no differences in clinical asthma scores or hospital discharge times between heliox and air groups.

In recent years, β2-agonist heliox-driven nebulization has gained popularity in ICU settings and emergency departments, where patients often experience severe asthma exacerbations. Heliox's physical properties allow for deeper aerosol penetration into distal airways and alveoli compared to oxygen or air, potentially improving bronchodilatation. Heliox aerosol delivery systems minimize particle-impaction drug loss, increasing the bronchodilator dose available to the lungs.

However, a significant challenge is that hypoxic patients may require a higher FiO_2 than the typically available 20% or 30% oxygen in heliox mixtures. Adding oxygen to increase the FiO_2 b reduces helium percentage, decreasing distal bronchodilator deposition. Despite this, low helium-oxygen mixtures may still benefit hypoxic patients. Radionuclide studies concluded that heliox is significantly more effective than air in depositing 3.6 μm particles in the alveolar regions, with a more pronounced effect in asthmatic subjects (See Figure 1) [9].

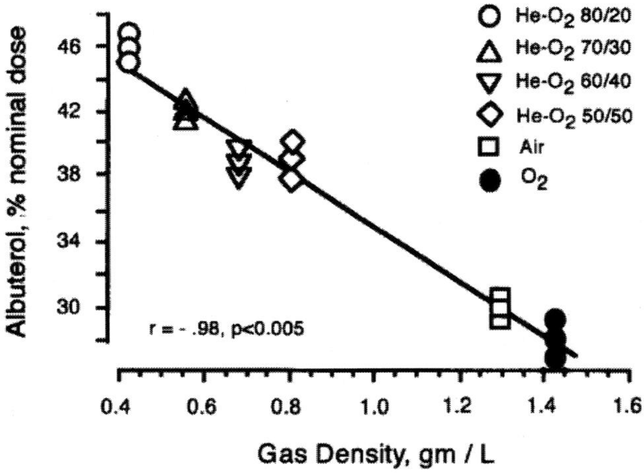

Figure 1. Gas density versus albuterol delivery.

Albuterol delivery is inversely related to gas density in the ventilator circuit [9]. Kim et al., [10] randomized subjects to receive continuous albuterol delivered by either 100% oxygen or heliox and observed improved pulmonary index scores and a higher likelihood hospital discharge within 12 hours in the heliox group. In 2010, another study noted a shorter emergency department stays for those receiving heliox-driven nebulized albuterol. A 2014 systematic review of heliox-driven nebulized β-agonist therapy reported increased peak expiratory flows and reduced hospital admissions for heliox compared with control groups, with a trend toward greater benefit in more severely affected subjects.

Given the conflicting results and study design heterogeneity, drawing firm conclusions about heliox use is challenging. While it is reasonable to initiate heliox for status asthmaticus patients in respiratory distress refractory to standard therapies, it should be discontinued if no clinical improvement occurs after a short therapeutic trial.

Heliox is commonly used in children with critical asthma. However. Lew et al., (2021) [6] conducted a multicenter retrospective study in 42 pediatric intensive care units and found that heliox prescribing for critical asthma declined over the last decade. In another study by the same authors, heliox was rarely used (2.5%) as adjunctive therapy for children with critical asthma and was not associated with mechanical ventilation or reduced ventilation duration.

Despite nearly nine decades of use, many reports on heliox are observational. Systemic reviews have generally failed to support heliox administration for moderate-to-severe acute asthma. A 2007Cochrane review of ten trials involving 544 patients concluded that heliox mixtures have no role in the initial treatment of acute asthma, although new evidence suggests possible benefits in patients with more severe obstruction, these data should be interpreted cautiously [10].

Heliox poses some risks, including the need for careful delivery monitoring, as some devices' flow meters cannot be calibrated for the different gas densities, leading to unreliable flow measurements. Prolonged heliox use may also hinder airway clearance by preventing turbulent flow during coughing. Furthermore, helium is a finite resource and should be used judiciously [11].

Guidelines, such as those from the Global Initiative for Asthma (GINA) [5] published in 2023, state that heliox has no role in routine care (evidence B), but may be considered for patients unresponsive to standard therapy, with availability, cost and technical issues taken into account. British guidelines [12] do not support heliox as a driving gas for nebulizers, as a breathing gas, or for artificial ventilation in adults with acute asthma. The main problem is that heliox requires the use of specifically designed or modified breathing circuits and ventilators. For them, heliox is not recommended for use in patients with acute asthma outside a clinical trial setting, and there is no evidence to support the use of heliox for the treatment of acute asthma in children. The guideline states: *"although the possibility of benefit exists in patients with more severe obstruction."*

In the "Guideline on Management of Acute Asthma Attacks in Children" by the Italian Society of Pediatrics (2022) [13], heliox (70/30) is recommended for severe asthma unresponsive to standard therapy, but not for mild-to-moderate cases. These recommendations are based on systematic reviews indicating insufficient data for routine heliox use in acute asthma, though it is considered safe, with some data suggesting potential benefits for patients with severely impaired lung function.

Despite the lack of concrete evidence, heliox should be considered in hospital protocols for acute asthma treatment in a particular set of patients, since there is a small number who do not respond to conventional therapy but still have respiratory muscle reserve.

At this time, heliox does not have a routine role in the acute management of asthma in emergency services, either in children or adults. However, in the case of patients who do not respond to treatment for a severe asthma attack, heliox is included_in the different guidelines as an adjunctive therapy, especially to improve the delivery of conventional inhaled therapy to the distal airways.

Conclusion

In conclusion, while heliox was first utilized for asthma treatment nearly 100 years ago based on its physical properties and the disease's pathophysiology, it is not a routine therapeutic option for asthma attacks. Instead, it remains a rescue option for severe crises unresponsive to corticosteroids or beta-agonists. Although its use has declined, international guidelines recognize heliox as an adjunct therapy, especially for delivering treatments to distal airways, while considering potential technical and economic challenges.

Key Messages

1. Heliox is a logical option in the treatment of acute asthma exacerbations based on the disease pathophysiology and helium's physical properties.
2. Recent studies indicate that heliox does not have a routine role in acute asthma management.
3. Heliox may be recommended for severe asthma unresponsive to standard therapy.
4. Heliox could serve as an adjunctive therapy, especially for improving the delivery of conventional inhaled therapy to distal airways in severe asthma cases.

5. Availability, cost and technical issues should be evaluated when considering heliox therapy.

References

[1] Wigmore T, Stachowski E. A review of the use of heliox in the critically ill. *Crit Care Resusc* 2006 Mar;8(1):64-72.

[2] Arias OJ, Salas FJ, Salas-Segura DA. Uso del heliox en las crisis asmáticas moderadas y severas en el Servicio de Emergencias del Hospital Rafael Ángel Calderón Guardia. Un estudio prospectivo. [Use of heliox in moderate and severe asthmatic attacks in the Emergency Department of the Rafael Ángel Calderón Guardia Hospital. A prospective study.] *Neumol Cir Torax* 2012;71(1):21-28.

[3] Beurskens, C. J., Wösten-van Asperen, R. M., Preckel, B., & Juffermans, N. P. (2015). The Potential of Heliox as a Therapy for Acute Respiratory Distress Syndrome in Adults and Children: A Descriptive Review. *Respiration* 89(2), 166–174.

[4] Hashemian SM, Fallahian F. The use of heliox in critical care. *Int J Crit Illn Inj Sci* 2014, Apr;4(2):138-42.

[5] Global initiative for asthma. Global Strategy for Asthma Management and Prevention 2023. July 2023. Available from: *www.ginasthma.org*.

[6] Lew. A, Russi. BW, Morrison. J, Anthony A. Sochet; Helium-Oxygen Mixture (Heliox) for Refractory Status Asthmaticus in the Intensive Care Unit: An Epidemiologic and Exploratory Comparative Analysis. *Pediatrics March* 2021, 147: 465–467.

[7] Carter ER, Webb CR, Moffitt DR. Evaluation of heliox in children hospitalized with acute severe asthma. A randomized crossover trial. *Chest* 1996 May;109(5):1256-61.

[8] Leatherman JW, Saavedra. R, Shapiro. R. Lack of Benefit of Heliox During Mechanical Ventilation of Subjects With Severe Air-Flow Obstruction. *Respiratory Care Apr* 2018, 63 (4) 375-379.

[9] Venkataraman S. T. Heliox During Mechanical Ventilation. *Respiratory Care Jun* 2006, 51 (6) 632-639.

[10] Kim IK, Phrampus E, Venkataraman S, Pitetti R, Saville A, Corcoran T, Gracely E, Funt N, Thompson A. Helium/oxygen-driven albuterol nebulization in the treatment of children with moderate to severe asthma exacerbations: a randomized, controlled trial. *Pediatrics* 2005 Nov;116(5):1127-33.

[11] Cruz, L, Ferreira. A. R, Coimbra. A, Castel-Branco M. G. Helium-oxygen mixtures and acute severe asthma. pages 216-217 (July - August 2009). DOI: 10.1016/j.aller. 2009.02.004.

[12] Scottish Intercollegiate Guidelines Network British Thoracic Society. *British guideline on the management of asthma.* July 2019.

[13] Indinnimeo L, Chiappini E, Miraglia Del Giudice M; Italian Panel for the management of acute asthma attack in children Roberto Bernardini. *Guideline on management of the acute asthma attack in children by Italian Society of Pediatrics. Ital J Pediatr* 2018 Apr 6;44(1):46.

Chapter 12

Heliox Therapy in Pulmonary Rehabilitation

Berkan Basançelebi[1,*]
Subhadeep Pal[2]
and Kadir İdin[3]
[1]Department of Electroneurophysiology, Vocational School,
Istanbul Medipol University, Istanbul, Turkey
[2]Department of Respiratory Care, Dr. D.Y. Patil School of Allied Health Sciences,
Pune, India
[3]Department of Anesthesiology and Reanimation, School of Medicine,
Istanbul Medipol University, Istanbul, Turkey

Abstract

Pulmonary rehabilitation (PR) plays a crucial role in managing chronic pulmonary disorders by aiming to alleviate symptoms and enhance patients' functional abilities. Although it is primarily utilized for treating chronic obstructive pulmonary disease, PR is now being used to address a variety of respiratory disorders. This comprehensive approach includes referral, evaluation, exercise training, and interdisciplinary education.

A recent addition to PR is the use of heliox, a mixture of helium and oxygen. Due to its lower density, heliox allows for smoother gas passage through the airways, reducing resistance and the work of breathing. This results in improved exercise performance, endurance, and peripheral muscle oxygenation, particularly in severe cases where exercise tolerance is significantly reduced.

However, despite its positive outcomes, there are challenges related to heliox delivery techniques and costs. Heliox serves as a temporary aid, providing relief while conventional medications take full effect.

* Corresponding Author's Email: berkanbasancelebi@gmail.com

In: Respiratory Care in Heliox Therapy Physiology and Technology
Editor: Antonio M. Esquinas
ISBN: 979-8-89530-385-6

Integrating heliox into PR, especially for patients with severe illness and limited exercise tolerance, has the potential to improve outcomes. Balancing its benefits against its limitations, and combining heliox with established treatments positions it as a valuable tool for improving the effectiveness of PR in chronic respiratory disorders.

Keywords: pulmonary rehabilitation, heliox, exercise training, aerosol medicine

Introduction

Pulmonary rehabilitation (PR) is a cornerstone in the management of chronic respiratory diseases, offering a multidisciplinary approach that combines exercise training, patient education, and behavioral strategies. Over the years, advancements in technology and innovative therapeutic interventions have enhanced the effectiveness of PR. One such promising innovation is the use of heliox—a helium-oxygen mixture known for its unique physical properties that facilitate smoother airflow through the airway [1, 2].

Heliox therapy has gained attention due to its potential to reduce airway resistance and alleviate the work of breathing in patients with chronic respiratory disorders, including chronic obstructive pulmonary disease (COPD), asthma, and interstitial lung disease. By lowering the density of inspired gas, heliox minimizes turbulence within the airways, improving gas exchange efficiency and enabling patients to engage in more intensive physical activity during rehabilitation sessions.

This chapter explores the integration of heliox therapy into pulmonary rehabilitation, focusing on its mechanisms of action, delivery methods, and clinical outcomes. While its benefits are promising, challenges such as cost, equipment availability, and proper administration protocols necessitate further exploration. Understanding the role of heliox in enhancing exercise capacity and overall quality of life in patients with chronic respiratory diseases will provide valuable insights into optimizing PR programs.

Definition of Pulmonary Rehabilitation

Pulmonary rehabilitation (PR) is a patient-centered medical approach crucial for treating chronic respiratory diseases. It involves a personalized, multidisciplinary program aimed at addressing both the physiological and psychological aspects of pulmonary conditions, with the goal of restoring patients to the highest possible functional capacity given their pulmonary limitations [1]. Patients with chronic obstructive pulmonary disease (COPD) often experience exertional dyspnea and fatigue, leading them to reduce their activity levels to avoid these symptoms. This reduction in activity can result in decreased confidence, depression, loss of employment or the ability to enjoy hobbies, and social isolation, all of which can lead to significant disability [2].

Decreased exercise capacity is directly related to dyspnea and exertional fatigue, and is further exacerbated by factors such as ventilatory constraints, pulmonary gas exchange mismatch, cardiac dysfunction, and peripheral muscle dysfunction, [3]. Skeletal muscle dysfunction is a major problem, leading to poor functional status, reduced balance, increased muscle fatiguability due to lower concentration of type 1 muscular fibers, and a decrease in the number and functionality of mitochondria [4-6].

Pulmonary rehabilitation is a well-established, clinically proven, and widely recognized therapeutic tool for improving the quality of life and functional capacity of patients with chronic pulmonary disorders. The primary goals of PR are to manage symptoms, particularly dyspnea, enhance functional exercise performance, reduce anxiety and depression, and improve health-related quality of life (HRQoL), thereby decreasing the frequency of hospitalizations [7]. PR has recently become the standard of care for various chronic respiratory conditions, including interstitial lung disease, thoracic restriction, bronchiectasis, pulmonary fibrosis, post-tuberculosis lung disease, cystic fibrosis, pulmonary hypertension, asthma, and during pre- and post-operative periods of lung resection, volume reduction or lung transplantation, and cancer [8-14].

Components of Pulmonary Rehabilitation

The main objectives of pulmonary rehabilitation are to reduce symptoms, particularly dyspnea, restore functional ability, and improve overall health. The clinical relevance of PR can be viewed from two perspectives: 'patient-centered,' focusing on the individual's respiratory condition, and 'society-centered,' addressing disease epidemiology and societal costs [15]. A PR program includes several comprehensive, evidence-based components that go beyond exercise training to include referrals, thorough patient assessment, education, and health-promoting behaviors [3].

Referral

Referral is a crucial initial step that remains an obstacle for many chronic respiratory disorders. [16]. While COPD patients are the traditional target population for PR, the program also benefits patients with non-COPD chronic respiratory diseases. Adaptations for non-COPD patients are necessary, such as excluding exercise-induced arrhythmias in pulmonary hypertension and providing education on airway clearance for patients with chronic suppurative lung disease. The most common clinical criterion for referral to PR is breathlessness on exertion, which can be clinically assessed using the Medical Research Council (MRC) Dyspnea Scale. This brief assessment scale helps identify individuals who may benefit from rehabilitation. The British Thoracic Society (BTS) recommends that patients with a 3-5 MRC dyspnea grade who are functionally limited by dyspnea should be referred for outpatient PR. Additionally, patients with a 2 MRC dyspnea grade who are functionally impaired by dyspnea should also be referred for PR. For those with less severe COPD and less breathlessness, adaptive and practical techniques to support exercise training should be considered. [17]. The point of referral provides an opportunity to assess the patient and explore their knowledge and perceptions of the program. It is also crucial to address any other comorbidities before starting the program.

Assessment

The evaluation should systematically address the inclusion and exclusion criteria while informing patients about the PR process. Outcome criteria aim to assess lung function, respiratory muscle strength, dyspnea, exercise performance, and general health status to guide both individual progress and program quality to achieve clinically significant improvements [18]. Pulmonary function testing, such as spirometry, is a key component of the rehabilitation physical examination. Spirometry is an affordable and widely available test, although it is effort-dependent, requiring the patient's knowledge, coordination, and cooperation with an experienced technician. It measures the forced expiratory volume in one second (FEV_1) and remains the gold standard for detecting airway obstruction. Recently, the forced expiratory volume at six seconds of exhalation (FEV_6) has been suggested as a more accurate diagnostic parameter for airway obstruction in COPD compared to vital capacity (VC) or forced vital capacity (FVC) [19].

Cardiopulmonary exercise testing (CPET) is considered the highest standard, measuring both objective cardiovascular responses and subjective factors such as dyspnea and leg fatigue. Common methods include the maximum incremental test and the constant work rate test. The maximum incremental test gradually increases the exercise intensity, to assess peak oxygen uptake and physiological responses at the limit of tolerance. This test also helps to assess trends, such as changes in minute ventilation relative to oxygen uptake (VO_2) or carbon dioxide production (VCO_2), which indicate ventilatory efficiency. The rate of change in VCO_2 compared to VO_2 is used to non-invasively determine the "anaerobic threshold." When performed on a bicycle ergometer, the rate of change in VO_2 relative to work rate helps to assess aerobic work efficiency [20].

During the constant work rate test, participants exercise at a constant fraction of their maximal or peak work rate (typically 50-80%) until they can no longer sustain the load. The duration of exercise is measured, and a steady state response—where energy demands are met by energy supply mechanisms—may or may not be reached. Even if a steady state is reached, it occurs over time and provides crucial information about the dynamic behavior of respiratory and cardiorespiratory functions and the body's ability to stabilize oxygen consumption [21].

In addition to CPET, other exercise tests, such as the six-minute walk test and the incremental and endurance shuttle walk tests, offer valuable insight into exercise tolerance, symptom severity, and arterial oxygen saturation levels [22-24]. Patient-reported outcomes, such as health-related quality of life (HRQoL), represent patients' perspectives on the mental, physical, and social impact of their condition. The Chronic Respiratory Disease Questionnaire (CRQ) and the St. George's Respiratory Questionnaire (SGRQ) are commonly used in randomized controlled trails to assess HRQoL in COPD patients. The CRQ consists of 20 items in four domains: dyspnea, fatigue, emotional function, and mastery, addressing symptoms and coping mechanisms. The SGRQ, originally consisting of 50 questions, evaluates symptoms, activity limitations, and the overall impact of respiratory disease on daily life [25].

The MRC Dyspnea Scale, the Baseline Dyspnea Index (BDI) and the Transition Dyspnea Index are used as patient-reported outcomes (PROs) to measure dyspnea and evaluate the effects of PR. Additionally, the Hospital Anxiety and Depression Scale (HADS) evaluates depression and anxiety symptoms and generates scores for each domain. Although not specifically designed for COPD patients, HADS is commonly used in COPD research studies.

Exercise Training

Among all the components of PR, exercise training is the one that is the best supported and the most critical. For individuals aiming to reduce dyspnea during exercise and increase exercise tolerance, lower limb endurance training is essential. This training should be personalized, developed throughout the program, and based on evaluations from exercise tests. Patients with COPD can benefit from these principles, as higher-intensity training generally has a greater physiological impact than lower-intensity training. The goal is to exercise at the highest intensity possible; however, many individuals are so limited by dyspnea that they often cannot achieve the required intensity.

The training schedule should outline the intensity, duration, and frequency of the exercise. Intensity can be prescribed based on the results from CPET performed on a treadmill or a cycle ergometer, or from various field tests. Exercise sessions should last between 20 to 30 minutes. Walking and cycling are both effective modalities for training.

Resistance training has received significant attention in recent years and is now recommended by international guidelines. This training typically involves gym equipment and lower limb exercises such as step-ups, sit-to-stands, and leg lifts, with the intensity gradually increasing throughout the program. Ankle weights may also be used to provide additional resistance. Upper limb resistance training with free weights should be included, along with unsupported physical activity.

Multidisciplinary Education and Multidisciplinary Team

Education is a logical and necessary component of PR, typically delivered in a group setting but supplemented with individual support and ongoing educational materials, such as device-based and online learning modules. The educational program often includes nutritional advice, relaxation and energy conservation techniques, guidelines for using oxygen therapy equipment, advice on sexual health, information on disease progression, medication management, and self-management strategies. This educational aspect enhances the patients' sense of well-being and empowers them to take a more active role in managing their illness. It has been shown to reduce resource use, particularly by decreasing unexpected hospital visits.

Patients learn coping and response skills from a multidisciplinary team, consisting primarily of respiratory therapists, physiotherapists, assistants, nurses, and physicians. Team members should possess basic and intermediate life support skills, with at least one member having advanced life support skills during training sessions.

The Novel Modality: Exercise Training with Heliox

In recent years, many modern techniques and innovations have emerged, with heliox (HeO_2) being one of the most prominent. Heliox was first introduced by Barach in the 1930s as an alternative to nitrogen as a carrier gas for oxygen [26]. The salient feature of helium is its low specific gravity, second only to hydrogen, which is highly combustible and thus unusable. The low specific gravity of helium results in a gas with low density, directly correlating with a higher flow rate. Combining helium and oxygen produces a gas (HeO_2) with a viscosity similar to air but with lower density [27].

Heliox reduces airway resistance to gas flow, enhancing ventilation in two important ways. First, inhaling heliox lowers the Reynolds number, converting turbulent flow into more efficient and smoother laminar flow. Second, due to its low density, HeO_2 reduces the pressure gradient required to achieve a specific amount of turbulent flow, theoretically minimizing the work of breathing. A notable characteristic of heliox is its physiological inactivity and insolubility in human tissues, with no bronchodilator or anti-inflammatory activity. Its primary benefit is as a temporary agent that works until conventional methods take effect [28]. The European Respiratory Society (ERS) suggests that HeO_2 breathing can improve exercise performance in COPD patients [29].

Before delving into the action of HeO_2, it is essential to understand how it helps reduce the clinical symptoms of COPD and other chronic respiratory diseases characterized by airflow limitation, dyspnea, and recurrent exacerbations. In severe cases, exercise ability is primarily hindered by increased ventilatory demand, lung dynamic hyperinflation, and reduced ventilatory capacity [30]. Airflow limitation is generally caused by narrowing of the airways or airway collapse, along with loss of elastic recoil, which are clinical features of emphysema. These factors lead to reduced expiratory flow reserve and increased dynamic hyperinflation. Higher dynamic hyperinflation increases work of breathing, resulting in dyspnea and decreased exercise tolerance.

Mode of Action

HeO_2, due to its lower density and high flow rate resulting from laminar flow in larger airways, reduces airflow resistance and decreases the work of breathing. It also increases expiratory flow, which reduces dynamic hyperinflation and improves gas exchange, leading to lower partial pressure of carbon dioxide in the arteries ($PaCO_2$) [31]. Reduced dynamic hyperinflation can further decrease work of breathing and, consequently, VCO_2 [28]. One of the most promising benefits of heliox administration is its ability to enhance exercise endurance time by improving ventilatory capacity. Heliox also improves peripheral muscle oxygenation, which aids in exercise training endurance, as reported by Chiappa et al., [32]. Additionally, patients feel less anxious, more confident, and more cooperative during exercises.

Equipment for HeO_2 Delivery

The administration of HeO_2 gas mixtures poses technical challenges for medical practitioners due to the lack of equipment specifically designed for this purpose. Some institutions have resorted to using 100% helium tanks and mixing in oxygen to achieve the desired HeO_2 concentration, which is a risky practice. If the oxygen source is accidentally disconnected, patients may receive pure helium, leading to oxygen deprivation and posing a significant risk to patient safety. This method is medically unsound and strictly prohibited.

Heliox, with its thermal conductivity six times that of air, can cause issues with heat and moisture loss during administration. Achieving appropriate heating and humidification of HeO_2 to prevent adverse outcomes is extremely difficult. Additionally, heliox's unique physical properties, such as increased heat conductivity, can interfere with the proper functioning of medical equipment. Therefore, clinicians must remain vigilant to ensure that HeO_2 treatment is delivered safely and effectively.

Delivery through Cylinder

In many healthcare institutions, HeO_2 therapy is typically administered through transportable gas cylinders at the patient's bedside. Most countries use "H" size cylinders containing either 80% helium and 20% oxygen (80:20) or 70% helium and 30% oxygen (70:30). Each tank, with approximately 4,500 liters of gas, provides about five hours of HeO_2 therapy, depending on the device and flow settings. Before initiating therapy, therapists must verify the tank contents and ensure a minimum 24-hours supply.

Special regulators and attachment equipment are required for HeO_2 therapy. While specific flow meters are available, some clinicians use air or oxygen flow meters for convenience, necessitating correction factors due to different flow rates. To ensure proper oxygen delivery and detect potential issues, HeO_2 delivery setups must include an oxygen analyzer with audible alerts. Clinicians may add 100% oxygen to the HeO_2 setup to accurately titrate oxygen and helium levels. Although medical gas blenders are available, they are often avoided due to HeO_2 waste from bleed flow. A closed HeO_2 delivery system is preferred for optimal patient benefit. When this is not feasible, a system with low room air entrainment that meets the patient's minute volume requirement is essential.

The non-rebreather valved reservoir oxygen mask is increasingly used for HeO_2 delivery, though challenges include ensuring a tight fit and preventing gas loss. A T-connector is used to bleed in 100% oxygen to accurately regulate HeO_2 concentration, improving control when using an 80/20 heliox tank as the primary mask supply. Although oxygen tents, hoods, and huts may appear to be closed-system options, they are ineffective for HeO_2 delivery. Ultimately, HeO_2 treatment requires careful administration, including precise equipment usage, concentration control, and attention to patient comfort and safety.

nCPAP Delivery

The nCPAP device can be used for administering HeO_2 treatment due to its closed gas delivery system, built-in alarms, active humidification, and capability to provide and monitor positive pressure. Chowdhury et al., found that HeO_2 administered via nCPAP reduced the work of breathing by 70-80% and increased tidal volume (V_T) by 30% compared to nitrox. The study concluded that using HeO_2 via nCPAP at a pressure of 4 cmH_2O is optimal for minimizing work of breathing and optimizing V_T [33].

Heliox and Aerosol Delivery

In pulmonary rehabilitation, patients often aerosolized medication to maintain bronchial muscle tone and prevent bronchoconstriction. HeO_2 can play a beneficial role when combined with therapeutic interventions such as bronchodilators. Although HeO_2 itself does not have bronchodilatory properties, it can enhance the effectiveness of aerosolized treatments by creating laminar flow through constricted airways and improving aerosol deposition by reducing impaction loss as the aerosol moves from larger to smaller airways [34].

Most commercially available nebulizers are not designed for use with HeO_2, so the flow must be adjusted to match the capabilities of the oxygen-driven system. It is recommended to use a large-volume nebulizer, which acts as a gas reservoir to meet the high inspiratory flow demands of patients. Some devices on the market combine large-volume nebulizers with both oxygen and heliox to achieve the required minute ventilation for continuous aerosol delivery. [35].

A newer approach involves using a high-flow nasal cannula (HFNC), which allows for effective delivery of aerosolized drugs with HeO_2. HFNC equipped with a vibrating mesh nebulizer is better tolerated by patients and includes a heated and humidified system (100% relative humidity). Studies have shown that aerosols can be efficiently delivered through HFNC at a minimum flow rate of 30 L/min [35]. Furthermore, aerosol delivery with HeO_2 through HFNC tends to improve the inhaled dose at mid and high flow rates compared to using 100% oxygen [36].

Conclusion

Pulmonary rehabilitation is a personalized medical approach that plays a crucial role in managing chronic respiratory diseases. It involves a multidisciplinary program tailored to each patient, addressing both the physiological and psychological aspects of their condition. The goal is to restore patients to the highest level of function possible given their pulmonary impairment. This approach integrates various innovative methods to provide optimal treatment. The addition of heliox therapy to pulmonary rehabilitation appears to be a promising development. Factors influencing the success of this combined treatment include selecting the appropriate modality, ensuring the correct interface, adjusting helium-oxygen concentrations, and managing aerosol use.

However, there is limited research on the effectiveness of combining PR with heliox therapy. Future studies are needed to comprehensively evaluate this approach. Furthermore, the cost-effectiveness of heliox therapy compared to conventional oxygen therapy remains uncertain. Given the higher cost of heliox, cost-effectiveness analyses targeting specific patient groups could provide valuable insights for healthcare providers.

Key Messages

1. Helium is four times more expensive than oxygen, therefore it should be reserved for patients with severe disease, poor exercise tolerance, and significant dyspnea.
2. The helium concentration should ideally be above 60%, and gas flows should meet or exceed the patient's inspiratory flow needs to prevent dilution of the HeO_2 mixture with ambient air.
3. Due to helium's high thermal conductivity, it can cause a decrease in body temperature when used for extended periods. Therefore, heat and humidity should be provided before administration.
4. A closed delivery system should be used to prevent leakage and maintain optimal gas delivery, maximizing the benefits of the treatment.
5. Administration is most effective with a non-rebreathing facemask, ensuring that the patient receives the highest possible concentration of heliox without mixing with ambient air.
6. Heliox therapy serves as a temporary solution until conventional therapies become effective or can be used alongside conventional treatments.
7. Patient tolerance and monitoring are crucial, especially when using aerosol delivery with medium and low flow through HFNC and vibrating mesh nebulizers in patients with distressed lungs.

References

[1] Nici L, Donner C, Wouters E, Zuwallack R, Ambrosino N, Bourbeau J, Carone M, Celli B, Engelen M, Fahy B, Garvey C, Goldstein R, Gosselink R, Lareau S, MacIntyre N, Maltais F, Morgan M, O'Donnell D, Prefault C, Reardon J, Rochester C, Schols A, Singh S, Troosters T; ATS/ERS Pulmonary Rehabilitation Writing Committee. American Thoracic Society/European Respiratory Society Statement on Pulmonary Rehabilitation. *Am J Respir Crit Care Med* 2006 Jun 15;173(12):1390–413.

[2] Evans RA, Goldstein RS. Pulmonary Rehabilitation. In: Jindal SK, editor. *Textbook of Pulmonary and Critical Care Medicine*. Dordrecht, Netherlands: Jaypee Brothers Medical Publishers; 2011.

[3] Spruit MA, Singh SJ, Garvey C, ZuWallack R, Nici L, Rochester C, Hill K, Holland AE, Lareau SC, Man WD, Pitta F, Sewell L, Raskin J, Bourbeau J, Crouch R, Franssen FM, Casaburi R, Vercoulen JH, Vogiatzis I, Gosselink R, Clini EM, Effing TW, Maltais F, van der Palen J, Troosters T, Janssen DJ, Collins E, Garcia-Aymerich J, Brooks D, Fahy BF, Puhan MA, Hoogendoorn M, Garrod R, Schols AM, Carlin B, Benzo R, Meek P, Morgan M, Rutten-van Mölken MP, Ries AL, Make B, Goldstein RS, Dowson CA, Brozek JL, Donner CF, Wouters EF; ATS/ERS Task Force on Pulmonary Rehabilitation. An Official American Thoracic Society/European Respiratory Society Statement: Key Concepts and Advances in Pulmonary Rehabilitation. *Am J Respir Crit Care Med* 2013 Oct 15;188(8):e13–64.

[4] Bui KL, Nyberg A, Rabinovich R, Saey D, Maltais F. The Relevance of Limb Muscle Dysfunction in Chronic Obstructive Pulmonary Disease. *Clin Chest Med* 2019 Jun;40(2):367–83.

[5] Panagiotou M, Polychronopoulos V, Strange C. Respiratory and lower limb muscle function in interstitial lung disease. *Chron Respir Dis* 2016 May;13(2):162–72.

[6] Maltais F, Decramer M, Casaburi R, Barreiro E, Burelle Y, Debigaré R, Dekhuijzen PN, Franssen F, Gayan-Ramirez G, Gea J, Gosker HR, Gosselink R, Hayot M, Hussain SN, Janssens W, Polkey MI, Roca J, Saey D, Schols AM, Spruit MA, Steiner M, Taivassalo T, Troosters T, Vogiatzis I, Wagner PD; ATS/ERS Ad Hoc Committee on Limb Muscle Dysfunction in COPD. An Official American Thoracic Society/European Respiratory Society Statement: Update on Limb Muscle Dysfunction in Chronic Obstructive Pulmonary Disease. *Am J Respir Crit Care Med* 2014 May 1;189(9):e15–62.

[7] Gordon CS, Waller JW, Cook RM, Cavalera SL, Lim WT, Osadnik CR. Effect of Pulmonary Rehabilitation on Symptoms of Anxiety and Depression in COPD. *Chest* 2019 Jul;156(1):80–91.

[8] Dowman L, Hill CJ, Holland AE. Pulmonary Rehabilitation for Interstitial Lung Disease. *Cochrane Database Syst Rev* 2014 Oct 6;(10):CD006322.

[9] Lee AL, Gordon CS, Osadnik CR. Exercise training for bronchiectasis. *Cochrane Database Syst Rev* 2021 Apr 6;4(4)

[10] Cavalheri V, Burtin C, Formico VR, Nonoyama ML, Jenkins S, Spruit MA, Hill K. Exercise training undertaken by people within 12 months of lung resection for non-small cell lung cancer. *Cochrane Database Syst Rev* 2019 Jun 17;6(6).

[11] Morris NR, Kermeen FD, Jones AW, Lee JY, Holland AE. Exercise-based rehabilitation programmes for pulmonary hypertension. Cochrane Airways Group, editor. *Cochrane Database Syst Rev* 2023 Mar 22: 2023(3).

[12] Cesario A, Ferri L, Galetta D, Pasqua F, Bonassi S, Clini E, Biscione G, Cardaci V, di Toro S, Zarzana A, Margaritora S, Piraino A, Russo P, Sterzi S, Granone P. Post-operative respiratory rehabilitation after lung resection for non-small cell lung cancer. *Lung Cancer* 2007 Aug;57(2):175–80.

[13] Talwar A, Sahni S, Verma S, Khan SZ, Dhar S, Kohn N. Exercise tolerance improves after pulmonary rehabilitation in pulmonary hypertension patients. *J Exerc Rehabil* 2017 Apr;13(2):214–7.

[14] Vagvolgyi A, Rozgonyi Z, Kerti M, Vadasz P, Varga J. Effectiveness of perioperative pulmonary rehabilitation in thoracic surgery. *J Thorac Dis* 2017 Jun;9(6):1584–91.

[15] Lusuardi M, Ambrosino N, Donner CF. Definition and Rationale for Pulmonary Rehabilitation. In: Donner CF, Ambrosino N, Goldstein R, editors. *Pulmonary rehabilitation.* New York, NY: Oxford University Press; 2005.

[16] Rochester CL, Vogiatzis I, Holland AE, Lareau SC, Marciniuk DD, Puhan MA, Spruit MA, Masefield S, Casaburi R, Clini EM, Crouch R, Garcia-Aymerich J, Garvey C, Goldstein RS, Hill K, Morgan M, Nici L, Pitta F, Ries AL, Singh SJ, Troosters T, Wijkstra PJ, Yawn BP, ZuWallack RL; ATS/ERS Task Force on Policy in Pulmonary Rehabilitation. An Official American Thoracic Society/European Respiratory Society Policy Statement: Enhancing Implementation, Use, and Delivery of Pulmonary Rehabilitation. *Am J Respir Crit Care Med* 2015 Dec 1;192(11):1373–86.

[17] Bolton CE, Bevan-Smith EF, Blakey JD, Crowe P, Elkin SL, Garrod R, Greening NJ, Heslop K, Hull JH, Man WD, Morgan MD, Proud D, Roberts CM, Sewell L, Singh SJ, Walker PP, Walmsley S; British Thoracic Society Pulmonary Rehabilitation Guideline Development Group; British Thoracic Society Standards of Care Committee. British Thoracic Society guideline on pulmonary rehabilitation in adults: accredited by NICE. *Thorax* 2013 Sep;68(Suppl 2):ii1–30.

[18] Brooks D, Sottana R, Bell B, Hanna M, Laframboise L, Selvanayagarajah S, Goldstein R. Characterization of Pulmonary Rehabilitation Programs in Canada in 2005. *Can Respir J* 2007;14(2):87–92.

[19] De Troyer A, Yernault JC. Inspiratory muscle force in normal subjects and patients with interstitial lung disease. *Thorax* 1980 Feb 1;35(2):92–100.

[20] Palange P, Ward SA, Carlsen KH, Casaburi R, Gallagher CG, Gosselink R, O'Donnell DE, Puente-Maestu L, Schols AM, Singh S, Whipp BJ. Recommendations on the use of exercise testing in clinical practice. *Eur Respir J* 2006 Sep 27;29(1):185–209.

[21] Radtke T, Crook S, Kaltsakas G, Louvaris Z, Berton D, Urquhart DS, Kampouras A, Rabinovich RA, Verges S, Kontopidis D, Boyd J, Tonia T, Langer D, De Brandt J, Goërtz YMJ, Burtin C, Spruit MA, Braeken DCW, Dacha S, Franssen FME, Laveneziana P, Eber E, Troosters T, Neder JA, Puhan MA, Casaburi R, Vogiatzis I, Hebestreit H. ERS statement on standardisation of cardiopulmonary exercise testing in chronic lung diseases. *Eur Respir Rev* 2019 Dec 31;28(154):180101.

[22] ATS Committee on Proficiency Standards for Clinical Pulmonary Function Laboratories. ATS Statement: Guidelines for the Six-Minute Walk Test. *Am J Respir Crit Care Med* 2002 Jul 1;166(1):111–7.

[23] Revill SM, Morgan MD, Singh SJ, Williams J, Hardman AE. The endurance shuttle walk: a new field test for the assessment of endurance capacity in chronic obstructive pulmonary disease. *Thorax* 1999 Mar;54(3):213–22.

[24] Singh SJ, Morgan MD, Scott S, Walters D, Hardman AE. Development of a shuttle walking test of disability in patients with chronic airways obstruction. *Thorax* 1992 Dec;47(12):1019–24.

[25] Jones PW, Quirk FH, Baveystock CM, Littlejohns P. A Self-complete Measure of Health Status for Chronic Airflow Limitation: The St. George's Respiratory Questionnaire. *Am Rev Respir Dis* 1992 Jun;145(6):1321–7.

[26] Barach AL. The Use Of Helium in the Treatment of Asthma and Obstructıve Lesions in The Larynx and Trachea. *Ann Intern Med* 1935 Dec 1;9(6):739.

[27] Browne-Heitschmidt MG, Cassidy JB. Heliox: a new treatment for life-threatening asthma. *Pediatr Nurs* 1997;23(5):479–82.

[28] [McGee DL, Wald DA, Hinchliffe S. Helium-oxygen therapy in the emergency department. *J Emerg Med* 1997;15(3):291–6.

[29] Palange P. Lighter than air: heliox breathing improves exercise tolerance in COPD. *Eur Respir Rev* 2010 Mar 1;19(115):1–3.

[30] O'Donnell DE. Hyperinflation, Dyspnea, and Exercise Intolerance in Chronic Obstructive Pulmonary Disease. *Proc Am Thorac Soc* 2006 Apr;3(2):180–4.

[31] Ball J, Rhodes A, Grounds R. A review of the use of helium in the treatment of acute respiratory failure. *Clin Intensive Care* 2001 Jun 1;12(3):105–13.

[32] Chiappa GR, Queiroga F, Meda E, Ferreira LF, Diefenthaeler F, Nunes M, Vaz MA, Machado MC, Nery LE, Neder JA. Heliox improves oxygen delivery and utilization during dynamic exercise in patients with chronic obstructive pulmonary disease. *Am J Respir Crit Care Med* 2009 Jun 1;179(11):1004–10.

[33] Chowdhury MM, Akhter R, Dixon PD, Habibi P. Heliox-Driven Cpap May Be More Effective Than Conventional Cpap In Reducing Work Of Breathing And Improving Tidal Volumes In Infant Respiratory Distress. *Chest* 2006 Oct 1;130(4):137S.

[34] Hess DR, Fink JB, Venkataraman ST, Kim IK, Myers TR, Tano BD. The history and physics of heliox. *Respir Care* 2006 Jun;51(6):608–12.

[35] Bhashyam AR, Wolf MT, Marcinkowski AL, Saville A, Thomas K, Carcillo JA, Corcoran TE. Aerosol delivery through nasal cannulas: an in vitro study. *J Aerosol Med Pulm Drug Deliv* 2008 Jun;21(2):181–8.

[36] Dailey PA, Harwood R, Walsh K, Fink JB, Thayer T, Gagnon G, Ari A. Aerosol Delivery Through Adult High Flow Nasal Cannula With Heliox and Oxygen. *Respir Care* 2017 Sep;62(9):1186–92.

Chapter 13

Heliox Therapy in Nasal High-Flow Oxygen

Sofia C. Silva[1,*], MD
and Antonio M. Esquinas[2], MD, PhD
[1]Pulmonology Department, Hospital Beatriz Ângelo, Portugal
[2]Intensive Care Unit, Hospital Morales Meseguer Molina Segura, Murcia, Spain

Abstract

Recently, high-flow oxygen therapy with nasal cannulas (HFNC) has gained considerable interest as an alternative to conventional oxygen therapy and non-invasive ventilation (NIV). HFNC delivers oxygen at elevated flow rates with humidified and heated gas, enhancing patient comfort. Despite the low certainty of evidence, HFNC is a valuable intervention for adults with acute respiratory failure, challenging the formulation of stronger recommendations, especially when compared to NIV.

Heliox therapy can be administered through high-flow oxygen systems. HFNC is better tolerated than NIV in awake patients, which has increased interest in understanding the use of heliox with this technology. The concurrent use of heliox aims to decrease airway resistance, particularly in obstructive diseases. However, clinical evidence supporting the simultaneous use of heliox with HFNC is limited, and its clinical application is restricted in cases of severe hypoxemia requiring high FiO_2.

Overall, HFNC and heliox therapy show promise for respiratory support, with HFNC emerging as a versatile and comfortable option. Given the limited evidence available, it is imperative to continue research to gain a

* Corresponding Author's Email: ana.campos.silva@hbeatrizangelo.pt

In: Respiratory Care in Heliox Therapy Physiology and Technology
Editor: Antonio M. Esquinas
ISBN: 979-8-89530-385-6

comprehensive understanding of the clinical impacts and optimal utilization of these therapies.

Keywords: high-flow oxygen, nasal cannula, heliox, aerosol therapy

Introduction

Recently, there has been a growing interest in high-flow oxygen therapy with nasal cannulas (HFNC) as an alternative to conventional oxygen therapy and non-invasive ventilation (NIV). HFNC is a form of respiratory support that delivers high flow rates of oxygen with humified and heated gas, maximizing patient comfort and tolerance. The gas flow typically ranges between 15 to 60 liters per minute in adults, and the fraction of inspired oxygen (FiO_2) can be adjusted by changing the oxygen concentration in the driving gas.

The effectiveness of HFNC therapy depends on delivering a low level of positive airway pressure, which is directly correlated with the flow rate. This mechanism facilitates a reduction in upper airway dead space, enhances pharyngeal dead space washout, diminishes nasopharyngeal resistance, and increases alveolar recruitment, ultimately decreasing the work of breathing. Additionally, this approach provides enhanced humidification, improves patient comfort and tolerance, allows for precise control of FiO_2, and supports better mucociliary clearance [1, 2].

Frat et al., conducted a randomized clinical trial involving 310 patients that failed to demonstrate the benefit of HFNC in reducing the intubation rate in patients with acute non-hypercapnic respiratory failure who did not have chronic respiratory pathology or cardiogenic etiology, compared to NIV. However, the study did find a reduction in 90-day ICU mortality when comparing HFNC to NIV [3].

The 2022 ERS clinical practice guidelines on HFNC in acute respiratory failure recommend using HFNC over NIV in cases of acute hypoxemic respiratory failure (conditional recommendation, very low certainty of evidence). However, for patients with COPD and acute hypercapnic respiratory failure, an ERS task force suggests a trial of NIV before considering HFNC (conditional recommendation, low certainty of evidence). Despite these recommendations, the overall level of evidence remains low, and further studies are needed to determine whether HFNC provides advantages over NIV in patients with acute respiratory failure [4]. It is crucial to closely monitor these patients, as delaying endotracheal intubation may worsen outcomes in those experiencing acute respiratory failure.

Nasal High Flow and Heliox Therapy

Heliox therapy relies on its concentration for effectiveness and is typically delivered through high-flow oxygen systems. In awake patients with acute respiratory distress, HFNC is better tolerated than non-invasive ventilation. With the development and increased availability of high-flow nasal cannula oxygen devices worldwide, it is important to understand the feasibility of heliox therapy delivery using these devices.

The use of low-density gases such as heliox is theorized to enhance oxygenation and reduce respiratory effort due to their lower flow resistance. Helium, being less dense than nitrogen found in ambient air, affects gas flow dynamics in the airways. When delivered through high-flow oxygen devices, heliox aims to benefit from helium's lower density to reduce airway resistance, potentially improving respiratory efficiency, especially in cases of obstruction or increased resistance [5].

Moore et al., conducted an in vitro study using an experimental model to test the effects of gas delivery via HFNC on upper airway pressure and gas washout. They concluded that heliox, compared to room air or oxygen, is expected to result in similar CO_2 clearance from the upper airway but markedly lower airway pressure [6, 7]. However, it is important to note that the use of heliox (usually in ratios of 80:20 or 70:30) limits its application in patients with severe hypoxemia requiring high FiO_2. Increasing the FiO_2 in the mixture raises the gas density delivered, thereby restricting potential benefits.

Clinical evidence supporting the benefits of heliox with HFNC in specific scenarios is limited, particularly in the adult population. In contrast, the pediatric population has several case reports and a few small trials that suggest potential benefits. A 2015 Cochrane review on the potential benefits of heliox therapy in conjunction with CPAP or HFNC in infants suggests it may reduce the length of treatment for respiratory distress due to bronchiolitis [8].

Heliox therapy can be delivered using widely employed high-flow oxygen therapy equipment, particularly devices like Vapotherm® (PrecisionFlow Heliox). Additionally, adaptations for devices such as Optiflow™ or Hamilton-H900 enable the effective delivery of heliox. These devices are designed to meet the specific requirements of patients who need high gas flow rates.

The use of HFNC with oxygen allows for the administration of aerosol therapy, such as salbutamol. The distal deposition of aerosols may be influenced by airflow and the diameter of the nasal cannulas. Further studies are needed to better understand the impact of these factors on therapeutic administration.

The utility of heliox therapy has been described as a method to improve the response to bronchodilator aerosols in both children and adults. This improvement is achieved by providing more laminar flow through constricted airways and reducing impactive losses of aerosol during transit from larger to smaller airways. Dailey et al., investigated these effects with HFNC in vitro. Although there was a trend towards improved inhaled dose at mid and high flows when delivering aerosols with heliox through HFNC compared to oxygen, the results failed to reach statistical significance [9, 10]. Based on the current evidence, it is not possible to recommend the use of aerosolized therapy with heliox in conjunction with HFNC.

Conclusion

HFNC and heliox therapy appear promising for respiratory support, with HFNC standing out as a versatile and more comfortable option for the patient. The potential advantages of heliox in decreasing airway resistance and enhancing respiratory efficiency —especially when administered through HFNC —are noteworthy. Nevertheless, clinical recommendations must be approached with caution due to the limited evidence available. Further research is necessary to understand the clinical impact of the lower FiO_2 limitations imposed by heliox therapy with HFNC.

Key Messages

1. There is a growing interest in high-flow oxygen therapy with nasal cannulas as an alternative to conventional oxygen and non-invasive ventilation (NIV) for acute respiratory failure.
2. HFNC presents several advantages, including providing some level of positive airway pressure, reducing dead space and respiratory effort, enhancing patient comfort, as well as enhancing mucociliary clearance through heated and humidified air.

3. Heliox therapy can be administered through HFNC devices in 80:20 or 70:30 ratios, which limits its use in patients requiring high FiO_2.

References

[1] Gotera, C., S. Díaz Lobato, T. Pinto, and J. C. Winck. "Clinical Evidence on High Flow Oxygen Therapy and Active Humidification in Adults." *Revista Portuguesa de Pneumologia* 2013,19,5: 217–27.

[2] Sztrymf, Benjamin, Jonathan Messika, Fabrice Bertrand, Dominique Hurel, Rusel Leon, Didier Dreyfuss, and Jean-Damien Ricard. "Beneficial Effects of Humidified High Flow Nasal Oxygen in Critical Care Patients: A Prospective Pilot Study." *Intensive Care Medicine* 2011: 37, no. 11 1780–86.

[3] Frat JP, Thille AW, Mercat A, Girault C, Ragot S, Perbet S, Prat G, Boulain T, Morawiec E, Cottereau A, Devaquet J, Nseir S, Razazi K, Mira JP, Argaud L, Chakarian JC, Ricard JD, Wittebole X, Chevalier S, Herbland A, Fartoukh M, Constantin JM, Tonnelier JM, Pierrot M, Mathonnet A, Béduneau G, Delétage-Métreau C, Richard JC, Brochard L, Robert R; FLORALI Study Group; REVA Network. "High-Flow Oxygen through Nasal Cannula in Acute Hypoxemic Respiratory Failure." *The New England Journal of Medicine* 2015 Jun 4;372(23): 2185-96.

[4] Oczkowski, Simon, Begüm Ergan, Lieuwe D. J. Bos, Michelle Chatwin, Miguel Ferrer, Cesare Gregoretti, Leo Heunks, Jean-Pierre Frat, Federico Longhini, Stefano Nava, Paolo Navalesi, Aylin Ozsancak Uğurlu, Lara Pisani, Teresa Renda, Arnaud W. Thille, João Carlos Winck, Wolfram Windisch, Thomy Tonia, Jeanette Boyd, Giovanni Sotgiu, Raffaele Scala. ERS Clinical Practice Guidelines: High-Flow Nasal Cannula in Acute Respiratory Failure. *Eur Respir J* 2022 Apr 14;59(4): 2101574.

[5] Hess, Dean R, Fink, James B, Venkataraman, Shekhar T, Kim, In K, Myers, Timothy R, Tano, Benoit D. The history and physics of heliox. *Respiratory Care* 2006; 51: 608–12.

[6] Moore, Charles P., Ira Katz, Georges Caillibotte, Warren H. Finlay, and Andrew Martin. "Correlation of High Flow Nasal Cannula Outlet Area with Gas Clearance and Pressure in Adult Upper Airway Replicas." *Clinical Biomechanics* 2019, Jun:66:66-73.

[7] Moore, C. P., I. M. Katz, M. Pichelin, G. Caillibotte, W. H. Finlay, and A. R. Martin. "High Flow Nasal Cannula: Influence of Gas Type and Flow Rate on Airway Pressure and CO2 Clearance in Adult Nasal Airway Replicas." *Clinical Biomechanics* 2019, 65, May: 73–80.

[8] Liet, Jean-Michel, Thierry Ducruet, Vineet Gupta, and Gilles Cambonie. "Heliox Inhalation Therapy for Bronchiolitis in Infants." *Cochrane Database of Systematic Reviews* 2015. September 18;2015 (9).

[9] O'Callaghan, Christopher, Judy White, Judith Jackson, David Crosby, Beatriz Dougill, and Hubert Bland. "The Effects of Heliox on the Output and Particle-Size

Distribution of Salbutamol Using Jet and Vibrating Mesh Nebulizers." *Journal of Aerosol Medicine* 2007: 20 Nº 4; 434–44.

[10] Dailey, Patricia A, Robert Harwood, Kyle Walsh, James B Fink, Tina Thayer, Greg Gagnon, and Arzu Ari. "Aerosol Delivery Through Adult High Flow Nasal Cannula with Heliox and Oxygen." *Respiratory Care* 2017, 62;9. 1186–92.

Chapter 14

Heliox in Non-Invasive Ventilation

Manjush Karthika*, PhD, PDF

Faculty of Medical and Health Sciences, Liwa College, Abu Dhabi, UAE

Abstract

Helium-oxygen (Heliox) mixtures have been used for decades in the management of diverse respiratory disorders ranging from acute upper airway to lower airway obstructions in neonatal, pediatric and adult populations. The delivery devices for heliox remain a topic of debate due to the physical properties of the gas. This chapter briefly discusses the physiology and utility of heliox when combined with non-invasive ventilation (NIV), summarizes the results of past and recent research related to this combination therapy, and outlines technical considerations relevant to its clinical application.

Keywords: helium, oxygen, heliox, non-invasive ventilation, airway resistance

Introduction

Non-invasive ventilation (NIV) has become a standard therapeutic approach in chronic obstructive pulmonary disease (COPD) patients experiencing acute exacerbations with acute respiratory failure [1]. Timely initiation of NIV drastically reduces the rate of endotracheal intubation, ventilator-associated pneumonia, length of stay in the intensive care unit (ICU), and associated

---

* Corresponding Author's Email: manjushnair@hotmail.com

In: Respiratory Care in Heliox Therapy Physiology and Technology
Editor: Antonio M. Esquinas
ISBN: 979-8-89530-385-6

mortality and morbidity [2]. Knowledge of the clinical and technical aspects of NIV—such as optimal indications, selection of interface, and improvements in patient-ventilator synchrony—is fundamental to its success, thereby minimizing the risk of complications [3]. Despite these factors, successful outcomes are possible with the addition of heliox to NIV, thereby preventing the need for invasive ventilation [4, 5].

Heliox, consisting of various concentrations of helium and oxygen, is an inert, nontoxic, and non-carcinogenic gas mixture known to have no lasting effects on any human organs [6]. The lower density of heliox (approximately six times lower than atmospheric air) is significant, as its inhalation results in significantly lower turbulence, particularly in the peripheral areas of the lungs. This facilitates a greater proportion of laminar flow and lowers overall airway resistance. The decreased turbulence can increase flow rates by up to 50% during the inhalation of heliox. This effect remains evident in cases of obstructive pulmonary diseases where airflow was restricted [7, 8]. The concept of combination therapy using NIV and heliox gained attention following a Swiss study [4] that reported positive outcomes in managing patients with acute exacerbation of chronic pulmonary diseases.

Helium-oxygen has complementary effects when used with NIV; indeed, the combination of heliox and NIV can even be considered synergistic. As a positive pressure therapy, NIV can help reduce the load on respiratory muscles, prevent or correct atelectasis, prevent airway collapse, and promote and facilitate the distribution of heliox throughout obstructed airways. Helium-oxygen can further reduce the work of breathing and improve CO_2 elimination. It can also provide higher expiratory flow than air-oxygen mixtures at the same pressure, which can help improve passive expiratory lung mechanics, reducing the risk of barotrauma due to gas trapping and thereby limiting any deleterious side effects from CPAP in obstructed airways [9].

Physiological Effects of Heliox-NIV

Heliox ventilation has been documented to diminish respiratory effort and reduce diaphragmatic load while demonstrating protective effects against atelectasis and airway collapse. While the patient is on heliox, it replaces the nitrogen and other gases, due to its low density, thereby reducing the Reynolds number (<2100), resulting in a laminar flow inside the airway. This reduces the pressure required to move gas through the airways, decreases airflow resistance and thereby reduces the work of breathing and dynamic hyperinflation. Additionally, it aids in the distribution of respiratory gases in narrow or constricted airways [10-12]. The use of helium-oxygen may enhance penetration into the peripheral regions of the lungs, thereby improving the ventilation/perfusion ratio. Moreover, heliox has the potential to enhance gas mixing in the alveoli, leading to improved carbon dioxide elimination [13, 14]. Studies have indicated that heliox ventilation results in a higher expiratory flow at the same pressure as a standard mixture [15-17]. This increased expiratory flow may facilitate passive exhalation, mitigating the risk of gas trapping and associated barotrauma [15, 18]. Several studies reported a decrease in oxygen demand with heliox ventilation. Heliox use was associated not only with a significant decrease in inflammatory mediators such as IL-8 and myeloperoxidase but also reduced diaphragmatic muscle injury score and better aeration of heliox-ventilated lungs [12, 19].

Clinical Applications of Heliox-NIV

Lower Airway Diseases

Heliox is indicated in cases of severe asthma exacerbations where conventional therapies may be insufficient. The use of heliox during NIV will optimize gas flow dynamics and alleviates respiratory distress. It is vital to recognize that heliox is not a universal solution but rather a targeted intervention for specific clinical scenarios. The administration of heliox during NIV involves standard modes like bilevel positive airway pressure (BiPAP) or continuous positive airway pressure (CPAP). Proper equipment and gas delivery systems are essential to ensure an optimal concentration of helium and oxygen as per clinical requirements. The amount of helium in the heliox mixture should be tailored to the patient's needs, considering factors such as age, respiratory rate, and severity of respiratory distress. Studies exploring the efficacy of heliox during NIV for asthma and chronic obstructive pulmonary disease (COPD) have demonstrated variable outcomes. While heliox has shown benefits in terms of improved respiratory mechanics and patient comfort, the evidence is not uniform across all patient populations. It appears to be more effective in certain subgroups, such as those with severe refractory asthma. Monitoring patient response and adjusting treatment accordingly are crucial aspects of using heliox during NIV. Before incorporating heliox into the management of asthma or COPD exacerbations, clinicians must consider the individual patient's condition, the severity of the exacerbation, and the response to initial therapies. Factors such as co-existing conditions, contraindications, and the availability of appropriate equipment also play a role in decision-making. Heliox should be viewed as an adjunctive therapy, not a replacement for standard treatments. Although heliox is generally considered safe, healthcare providers must be aware of potential complications. Helium is an inert gas, and the risk of barotrauma may be reduced compared to other gases. Nevertheless, careful monitoring for adverse effects, including changes in respiratory status, is essential. In addition, the unique properties of helium may affect the accuracy of certain medical devices, and adjustments may be necessary. Research on the use of heliox with NIV for asthma is evolving. A Cochrane review has explored the role of heliox in non-intubated acute asthma patients, indicating potential benefits in terms of improved outcomes [20]. However, further high-quality studies are needed to establish a more comprehensive understanding of combining heliox with NIV in asthma management. The use of heliox in combination with NIV in patients presenting with COPD exacerbations is observed to have promising outcomes [21]. Combining heliox with NIV effectively alleviates respiratory effort in COPD exacerbations. Jolliet et al., proposed that integrating heliox with NIV would aid decompensating COPD patients. Their study concluded that this combination reduced both $PaCO_2$ and dyspnea levels in the patients [4]. In their subsequent prospective, randomized, multicenter study, they also concluded that heliox-NIV reduced post-ICU stay by approximately 6 days and overall hospital costs [22]. Existing literature agrees that heliox is safe with no adverse effects reported. The improved flow properties and higher CO_2 diffusion coefficient of heliox make it a potential alternative in the management of severe airway obstruction [15].

Upper Airway Obstruction

Heliox has been promoted as an adjunctive therapy for severe upper airway obstruction in pediatric patients [23]. Combined therapy with CPAP has also been proven effective [24]; while heliox provides the benefits mentioned earlier, NIV decreases the workload on the inspiratory muscles, prevents airway collapse and promotes heliox distribution [24-26]. Heliox appears to be a reasonable option in severe respiratory distress that results from upper airway obstruction [27]. The gas mixture may allow clinicians to "buy time" while awaiting treatment aimed at alleviating the obstruction. Helium has no curative action in upper airway obstruction [28, 29], and in a randomized controlled study [30] no difference was found between heliox and racemic epinephrine in alleviating symptoms in children with moderate upper airway obstruction. However, heliox has been found beneficial in improving patient outcomes and comfort while breathing, especially when treating conditions like croup, epiglottitis, and laryngitis [18, 31, 32]. Heliox delivered via helmet interface CPAP mode is proposed as an alternative to avoid endotracheal intubation while managing severe upper airway obstruction in infants who are unresponsive to standard therapy [33].

Post-Extubation Respiratory Distress

In the context of post-extubation distress, the application of heliox in conjunction with NIV emerges as a promising strategy to alleviate respiratory challenges. Post-extubation distress often involves increased work of breathing and respiratory discomfort in patients transitioning from mechanical ventilation. Heliox, with its lower density, facilitates improved gas flow and can reduce airway resistance, making it a valuable adjunct to NIV interventions. By employing heliox in post-extubation NIV, clinicians may enhance patient comfort and respiratory mechanics, ultimately aiding in the prevention or management of respiratory failure. Many existing studies support the use of NIV following the post-extubation period in patients who are experiencing or are prone to developing distress [34, 35], and the addition of heliox is likely to have potential benefits in reducing post-extubation distress. This approach represents a nuanced therapeutic option, offering clinicians a means to optimize respiratory support and improve outcomes in patients facing challenges after extubation.

Respiratory Distress Syndrome

Colnaghi et al., conducted a randomized controlled trial involving preterm infants with respiratory distress syndrome (RDS), comparing nasal continuous positive airway pressure (nCPAP) with a helium-oxygen mixture (4:1 He:O2) to medical air. The use of heliox in this study significantly reduced the need for mechanical ventilation and surfactant administration [36]. Another randomized controlled trial from China in 2014 investigated the outcomes of nasal intermittent positive pressure ventilation with heliox in neonates with

RDS, revealing shorter ventilation duration and improved carbon dioxide removal [37]. In a recent study by Neumann-Klimasinska et al., a helium-oxygen mixture was applied in conjunction with non-invasive neurally adjusted ventilatory assist (NIV-NAVA) either as the primary respiratory support or post-extubation. This approach demonstrated a prompt and substantial reduction in Edi, indicating reduced respiratory effort. Additionally, a decrease in respiratory rate and peak inspiratory pressure was observed [10]. In a systematic review and meta-analysis conducted in 2016, the effects of heliox-NIV were evaluated in preterm infants with RDS. The analysis comprised 2 randomized controlled trials and 1 quasi-randomized controlled trial, involving a total of 123 neonates. Heliox-NIV, when compared to a standard gas mixture, significantly reduced the incidence of intubation. Its application was also linked to a decrease in $PaCO_2$ levels and a lower frequency of surfactant administration. No significant differences were observed in other secondary outcomes, including the duration of NIV and hospitalization, as well as the incidence of bronchopulmonary dysplasia (BPD), patent ductus arteriosus, necrotizing enterocolitis, intraventricular hemorrhage, periventricular leukomalacia, and mortality. NIV with heliox is also found useful in decreasing the incidence of intubation in preterm infants suffering from RDS [38].

Bronchopulmonary Dysplasia

Heliox has been used in infants diagnosed with established bronchopulmonary dysplasia (BPD), either non-invasively or via an endotracheal tube. In a study conducted by Wolfson et al., heliox mixtures with ratios of 80:20 and 70:30 were administered to spontaneously breathing BPD patients via face masks while monitoring pulmonary function parameters. Clinical assessments showed that infants breathing heliox exhibited more regular and less effortful breathing compared to those using air-oxygen mixtures. These findings were consistent with measured outcomes, indicating a significant decrease in both the work of breathing and pulmonary resistance [12]. Notably, the positive effects of heliox were evident in infants with BPD when heliox was administered with positive pressure via NIV [39, 40].

Heliox-NIV in Pediatric Patients

Currently there are no firmly established indications for the use of heliox with NIV in the pediatric population. However, based on available literature, a list of potential indications for heliox in combination with NIV for pediatric patients are summarized in Table 1 [18]. This list derives from the physical properties of heliox, alongside findings from experimental studies and clinical reports involving adult patients. In pediatric patients on heliox therapy but not achieving sufficient oxygenation levels, the application of NIV can improve alveolar recruitment and oxygenation, allowing for a reduction in FiO_2 and an increase in the fraction of helium. In cases where patients are already on NIV but demonstrate inadequate ventilation (as indicated by pH/pCO_2 levels, dyspnea, or clinical scores), heliox can enhance alveolar ventilation and CO_2 elimination without requiring further adjustments to NIV parameters.

Table 1. Indications of heliox with NIV in the pediatric population

Children already receiving heliox with inadequate oxygenation:
Not meeting their oxygenation goals.
FiO_2 requirement is ≥ 0.40.
Children already receiving NIV with inadequate ventilation:
Ventilation level is inadequate according to pH/pCO_2.
Require high or increasing pressure levels (PIP/IPAP)
Show insufficient improvement or worsening in dyspnea
Show insufficient improvement or worsening in clinical respiratory score.
Children receiving NIV whose underlying pathology or illness requires a protective ventilatory strategy:
Lowest possible pressure/volume swing (amplitude/IPAP-EPAP) for achieving a target pH/CO2 level.

Equipment and Technical Aspects

Heliox is usually delivered through interfaces such as non-rebreather masks or positive pressure devices. When delivering heliox via NIV, clinicians should adhere to specific technical consideration as:

1. Ensure all circuit connections are properly made and the ventilator is set to deliver a gas mixture of helium and oxygen, with sensors calibrated according to technical recommendations.

2. Set FiO_2 at 100% when connected to the heliox blending source to ensure accurate delivery, as the ventilator will utilize all gas from the connected source.
3. Once the other parameters are set, set the alarms correctly. A low-pressure alarm may be triggered during heliox use, as helium is a lighter gas, which can lead to detected pressures being lower. The pressures decrease by half when heliox is used.
4. Monitor the rate of emptying of gas tanks or cylinders while delivering heliox to the patient. Using a single-limb circuit may cause cylinders to empty faster due to leaks through the exhalation port; thus, backup cylinders are recommended.
5. An appropriate gas blender is required for Heliox delivery. Since flowmeters are not calibrated for heliox, a conversion factor must be used to determine the actual flow. The conversion factors are:
   a) 80-20 mixture: 1.8
   b) 70-30 mixture: 1.6
   c) 60-40 mixture: 1.4 [41].

Conclusion

In conclusion, heliox used in conjunction with NIV presents a promising option for managing various respiratory conditions, particularly those characterized by airway obstruction. Although literature is still limited, this combination therapy has shown efficacy in conditions such as asthma and COPD exacerbations, as well as neonatal presentations. However, further research is needed to better understand its optimal utilization, potential benefits, long-term effects, and applicability across different patient populations.

Key Messages

1. Heliox, with its lower density, facilitates better gas flow through constricted airways, enhancing oxygenation and CO_2 elimination in patients who are on NIV.

2. By decreasing airway resistance, heliox decreases the work of breathing, which is especially beneficial in conditions like asthma and COPD.
3. Heliox therapy often improves patient comfort while on NIV due to smoother flow dynamics, reducing dyspnea and promoting adherence to treatment.
4. While heliox offers promising benefits, its efficacy may vary depending on the patient's underlying condition, severity of respiratory distress, and the specific ventilator settings. Clinicians must carefully assess each case to determine the appropriateness of heliox therapy.
5. Continued research is essential to further elucidate the optimal use of heliox in NIV, refine delivery methods, identify patient populations likely to benefit, and explore novel applications in respiratory care.

References

[1] Davidson AC, Banham S, Elliott M, Kennedy D, Gelder C, Glossop A, Church AC, Creagh-Brown B, Dodd JW, Felton T, Foëx B, Mansfield L, McDonnell L, Parker R, Patterson CM, Sovani M, Thomas L; BTS Standards of Care Committee Member, British Thoracic Society/Intensive Care Society Acute Hypercapnic Respiratory Failure Guideline Development Group, On behalf of the British Thoracic Society Standards of Care Committee. BTS/ICS guideline for the ventilatory management of acute hypercapnic respiratory failure in adults. *Thorax* 2016;71: ii1–ii35.

[2] Chandra D, Stamm JA, Taylor B, Ramos RM, Satterwhite L, Krishnan JA, Mannino D, Sciurba FC, Holguín F. Outcomes of noninvasive ventilation for acute exacerbations of chronic obstructive pulmonary disease in the United States, 1998-2008. *Am J Respir Crit Care Med* 2012;185(2):152–9.

[3] Stefan MS, Nathanson BH, Higgins TL, Steingrub JS, Lagu T, Rothberg MB, Lindenauer PK. Comparative Effectiveness of Noninvasive and Invasive Ventilation in Critically Ill Patients With Acute Exacerbation of Chronic Obstructive Pulmonary Disease. *Crit Care Med* 2015;43(7):1386–94.

[4] Jolliet P, Tassaux D, Thouret JM, Chevrolet JC. Beneficial effects of helium:oxygen versus air:oxygen noninvasive pressure support in patients with decompensated chronic obstructive pulmonary disease. *Crit Care Med* 1999;27(11):2422–9.

[5] Laden G. Helium/oxygen and severe COPD. *Lancet* 2001;357(9255):559–60.

[6] Harris PD, Barnes R. The uses of helium and xenon in current clinical practice. *Anaesthesia* 2008; 63:284–93.

[7] Hunt T, Williams MT, Frith P, Schembri D. Heliox, dyspnoea and exercise in COPD. *Eur Respir Rev* 2010; 19:30–8.

[8] Eves ND, Ford GT. Helium-oxygen: A versatile therapy to "lighten the load" of chronic obstructive pulmonary disease. *Respir Med COPD Update* 2007; 3:87–94.

[9] Martinon-Torres F. Non-invasive ventilation with heliox. In: Medina A, Pons M, Martinon-Torres F, editors. Non-invasive ventilation in Pediatrics. 2nd ed. Madrid: Ergon; 2009. p. 99-106.

[10] Neumann-Klimasińska N, Merritt TA, Beck J, Miechowicz I, Szymankiewicz-Breborowicz M, Szczapa T. Effects of heliox and non-invasive neurally adjusted ventilatory assist (NIV-NAVA) in preterm infants. *Sci Rep* 2021: 11:15778.

[11] Migliori C, Gancia P, Garzoli E, Spinoni V, Chirico G. The Effects of helium/oxygen mixture (heliox) before and after extubation in long-term mechanically ventilated very low birth weight infants. *Pediatrics* 2009; 123:1524–8.

[12] Wolfson MR, Bhutani VK, Shaffer TH, Bowen FW, Jr. Mechanics and energetics of breathing helium in infants with bronchopulmonary dysplasia. *J Pediatr* 1984; 104:752–7.

[13] Frazier MD, Cheifetz IM. The role of heliox in paediatric respiratory disease. *Paediatr Respir Rev* 2010; 11:46–53.

[14] Nawab US, Touch SM, Irwin-Sherman T, Blackson TJ, Greenspan JS, Zhu G, Shaffer TH, Wolfson MR. Heliox attenuates lung inflammation and structural alterations in acute lung injury. *Pediatr Pulmonol* 2005; 40:524–32.

[15] Hashemian SM. Fallahian F. The use of heliox in critical care. *Int J Crit Illn Inj Sci* 2014; 4:138–42.

[16] Szczapa T, Gadzinowski J, Moczko J. Heliox augmented mechanical ventilation in the treatment of premature infants with respiratory distress syndrome. *Ginekol Pol* 2014; 85:939–43.

[17] Szczapa T, Gadzinowski J, Moczko J, Allen Merritt T. Heliox for mechanically ventilated newborns with bronchopulmonary dysplasia. *Arch Dis Child Fetal Neonatal Ed* 2014; 99: F128–33.

[18] Martinón-Torres F. Noninvasive ventilation with helium-oxygen in children. *J Crit Care* 2012; 27:220. e1–e2209.

[19] Elleau C, Galperine RI, Guenard H, Demarquez JL. Helium-oxygen mixture in respiratory distress syndrome: a double-blind study. *J Pediatr* 1993; 122:132–6.

[20] Rodrigo G, Pollack C, Rodrigo C, Rowe BH. Heliox for nonintubated acute asthma patients. *Cochrane Database Syst Rev* 2006;2006(4):CD002884.

[21] Mutlu GM, Budinger GR. Not much turbulence: Addition of heliox to noninvasive ventilation fails to improve outcomes in patients with exacerbations of chronic obstructive pulmonary disease. *Crit Care Med* 2010; 38:319–20.

[22] Jolliet P, Tassaux D, Roeseler J, Burdet L, Broccard A, D'Hoore W, Borst F, Reynaert M, Schaller MD, Chevrolet JC. Helium-oxygen versus air-oxygen noninvasive pressure support in decompensated chronic obstructive disease: a prospective, multicenter study. *Crit Care Med* 2003;31(3):878–84.

[23] Cambonie G, Milesi C, Fournier-Favre S, Counil F, Jaber S, Picaud JC, Matecki S. Clinical effects of heliox administration for acute bronchiolitis in young infants. *Chest* 2006; 129: 676-82.

[24] Mayordomo-Colunga J, Medina A, Rey C, Concha A, Los Arcos M, Menéndez S. Helmet-delivered continuous positive airway pressure with heliox in respiratory syncytial virus bronchiolitis. *Acta Paediatric* 2010; 99: 308-11.

[25] Antonelli M, Conti G, Pelosi P, Gregoretti C, Pennisi MA, Costa R, Severgnini P, Chiaranda M, Proietti R. New treatment of acute hypoxemic respiratory failure: noninvasive pressure support ventilation delivered by helmet – a pilot controlled trial. *Crit Care Med* 2002; 30: 602–8.

[26] Martinon-Torres F, Rodriguez-Nunez A, Martinon-Sanchez JM. Nasal continuous positive airway pressure with heliox in infants with acute bronchiolitis. *Respir Med* 2006; 100: 1458-62.

[27] Manthous CA, Morgan S, Pohlman A, Hall JB. Heliox in the treatment of airflow obstruction. *Respir Care* 1997; 42: 1034-42.

[28] Jolliet P, Tassaux D, Chevrolet J. Beneficial effects of helium-oxygen mixtures in acute respiratory failure. In: Yearbook of Intensive Care and Emergency Medicine. Edited by Vincent J. Berlin: Springer Verlag; 1999, 244-251.

[29] Boorstein JM, Boorstein SM, Humphries GN, Johnston CC. Using helium-oxygen mixtures in the emergency management of acute upper airway obstruction. *Ann Emerg Med* 1989; 18: 688-90.

[30] Weber JE, Chudnofsky CR, Younger JG, Larkin GL, Boczar M, Wilkerson MD, Zuriekat GY, Nolan B, Eicke DM. A randomized comparison of helium-oxygen mixture (heliox) and racemic epinephrine for the treatment of moderate to severe croup. *Pediatrics* 2001; 107: E96.

[31] Hess DR, Fink JB, Venkataraman ST, Kim IK, Myers TR, Tano BD. The history and physics of heliox. *Respir Care* 2006;51(6):608-12.

[32] Gupta VK, Cheifetz IM. Heliox administration in the pediatric intensive care unit: an evidence-based review. *Pediatr Crit Care Med* 2005;6(2):204-11.

[33] Vivanco-Allende A, Mayordomo-Colunga J, Coca-Pelaz A, Rey C, Medina A. Helmet-delivered heliox-CPAP in severe upper airway obstruction caused by PHACES syndrome. *Pediatr Pulmonol* 2011;46(3):306-8.

[34] Hernández G, Paredes I, Moran F, Buj M, Colinas L, Rodríguez ML, Velasco A, Rodríguez P, Pérez-Pedrero MJ, Suarez-Sipmann F, Canabal A, Cuena R, Blanch L, Roca O. Effect of postextubation noninvasive ventilation with active humidification vs high-flow nasal cannula on reintubation in patients at very high risk for extubation failure: a randomized trial. *Intensive Care Med* 2022;48(12):1751-59.

[35] Singh L. Role of Prophylactic Noninvasive Ventilation in Patients at High Risk of Extubation Failure. *Indian J Crit Care Med* 2020;24(12):1158-60.

[36] Colnaghi M, Pierro M, Migliori C, Ciralli F, Matassa PG, Vendettuoli V, Mercadante D, Consonni D, Mosca F. Nasal continuous positive airway pressure with heliox in preterm infants with respiratory distress syndrome. *Pediatrics* 2012; 129: e333–8.

[37] Li X, Shen J, Zhao J, Tang S, Shi Y. Nasal intermittent positive pressure ventilation with heliox in premature infants with respiratory distress syndrome: a randomized controlled trial. *Indian Pediatr* 2014: 51:900–2.

[38] Long C, Li W, Wanwei L, Jie L, Yuan S. Noninvasive ventilation with heliox for respiratory distress syndrome in preterm infant: a systematic review and meta-analysis. *Can Respir J* 2016; 2016:9092871.

[39] de Gamarra E, Moriette G, Farhat M, Walti H. Heliox tolerance in spontaneously breathing neonates with bronchopulmonary dysplasia. *Biol Neonate* 1998; 74: 193–9.

[40] Butt WW, Koren G, England S, Shear N, Whyte H, Bryan C, Swyer PR. Hypoxia associated with helium-oxygen therapy in neonates. *J Pediatr* 1985; 106:474–7.

[41] Fink J. Opportunities and Risks of Using Heliox in Your Clinical Practice. *Respiratory Care* 2006;51(6):651–60.

Chapter 15

Heliox Therapy in Invasive Mechanical Ventilation. Clinical Results

Salvatore Notaro*, MD
Andrea Imparato, MD
and Eugenio Piscitelli, MD
Department of critical care, Intensive care Unite and ECMO,
Monaldi - Colli Hospital, Naples, Italy

Abstract

Invasive ventilation is defined as the delivery of positive pressure to the lungs via an endotracheal or tracheostomy tube. It provides life-saving treatment for critically ill patients by supporting lung function, resting respiratory muscles, and allowing for adequate gas exchange.
Through this process, a mixture of air or oxygen and other gases, such as helium, is introduced into the airways and then flows into the alveoli.
Helium (He) is a chemical element and an inert gas that belongs to the class of noble gases on the periodic table. It is the second lightest element, with only hydrogen being lighter. Helium has low solubility and different density and viscosity properties compared to other gases. Its first clinical application dates back to the 1930s. Over the years, the impact of using heliox on various pathological conditions in both the upper and lower airways has been studied. These properties could be clinically useful in critical care settings, especially for patients with upper to more distal airway obstruction. Despite decades of use, providing firm clinical recommendations for its use in this setting remains difficult. The physiological benefits of breathing a helium-oxygen mixture in acute

* Corresponding Author's E-email: notaro@hotmail.it

In: Respiratory Care in Heliox Therapy Physiclogy and Technology
Editor: Antonio M. Esquinas
ISBN: 979-8-89530-385-6

severe asthma have been demonstrated. During upper airway obstructions, the flow in the airways changes from laminar to turbulent, resulting in increased resistance and increased work of breathing with muscle fatigue and easy exhaustion, which causes respiratory failure requiring orotracheal intubation and mechanical ventilation. Therefore, a less dense gas, such as a helium-oxygen mixture, flows better under turbulent conditions. Numerous studies have shown significant clinical benefits in lung function and respiratory mechanics for patients using ventilators. This leads to better delivery of inhaled medications, reducing mortality rates, aiding in the transition from invasive ventilation to regular breathing, and shortening hospital stays. The use of Heliox is recommended for patients with lower airway obstruction.

Keywords: helium-oxygen, heliox, mechanical ventilation, airway obstruction, asthma

Introduction

Invasive mechanical ventilation is defined as the delivery of positive pressure to the lungs via an endotracheal or tracheostomy tube. It includes an endotracheal tube (ETT) and a mechanical ventilator (MV). In addition to serving as a conduit for delivery of mechanical breaths, the ETT protects the airway, allows suction of secretions, and facilitates selected procedures, including bronchoscopy. The purpose of mechanical ventilation is to support lung function in critically ill patients and those undergoing general anesthesia. It allows the respiratory muscles to rest and facilitates adequate gas exchange. During this process, a blend of air or oxygen with other gases like helium is delivered into the airways and then transfers into the alveoli. This action inflates the lungs and raises the intra-alveolar pressure. When a flow or pressure termination signal interrupts the intake of air into the airways, the pressure in the central airways decreases. This causes expiration to occur passively, with air flowing from the higher pressure alveoli to the lower pressure central airways. By using mechanical ventilation (MV), it is possible to increase alveolar ventilation, which facilitates pulmonary gas exchange. This correction of hypoxemia increases PaO2 and oxygen transport (DO2) while decreasing systemic or myocardial oxygen consumption (VO2) [1]. Thanks to mechanical ventilation (MV), patients in acute respiratory acidosis are able to quickly correct their academia by achieving a normal arterial PCO2. MV also helps to treat and prevent atelectasis by inflating the lungs during inhalation, which has positive effects on oxygenation, compliance, and pulmonary defense mechanisms. These effects reduce the work of breathing, alleviate muscle fatigue, and decrease patient discomfort, allowing for sedation and neuromuscular block. Overall, mechanical ventilation is a lifesaving treatment for many critically ill patients with various pathological conditions [2]. Among the available mechanical ventilation mixtures, heliox is a blend of oxygen and helium. Elemental helium (He) is an inert gas in Group 18 (noble gases) of the periodic table. It's the second lightest element after hydrogen, and is colorless, odorless, and tasteless. Helium has the lowest boiling and freezing points of any known substance. Under normal atmospheric pressure, helium cannot be solidified; it requires a pressure of 25 atmospheres at a temperature of 1 K (-272°C. or -458°F) to convert it to its solid form. Helium makes up about 23 percent of the mass of the universe, second only to hydrogen. It's concentrated in high amounts in stars, where it is synthesized from hydrogen by nuclear fusion. Helium can be found in Earth's atmosphere or it can be extracted from cleveite, a mineral found in uranium deposits. It was discovered in 1868 by the French astronomer Janssen, who observed a bright yellow line in the sun's atmosphere during a total solar eclipse in India. The gas was named later that year when the English astronomer Lockyer observed it in the solar spectrum. He concluded that it was an element in the sun not found on Earth and named it after the Greek word for sun, helios. Initially, it was a dubious honor, as many colleagues doubted that it could be a new element and ridiculed his conclusions. Others thought that helium could exist only in the sun. In 1882, the Italian physicist Luigi Palmieri was analyzing lava from Mount Vesuvius when he noticed that same telltale yellow spectral line in his data — the first indication of helium on Earth. It would be another 12 years before the Scottish chemist William Ramsey found further experimental evidence of this new element. Once its physical properties were delineated, many useful applications for helium became apparent [3]. The combination of Helium and oxygen is a mixture called Heliox. First described in 1934, A. L. Barach tested various mixtures of helium and oxygen, finding benefit across a range of concentrations in asthmatic patients and infants with airway obstruction. [4]. The physical properties of helium, such as its low density and molecular weight, allow it to flow through airways with less turbulence than air or O2. Its incombustibility became especially desirable after the Hindenburg disaster in 1936, following which helium quickly replaced hydrogen as the gas of choice for dirigibles. The Medical Department of the US Navy-NEDU (Navy Experimental Diving Unit) was the first organization to use helium in a clinical setting. In May

1939, during the dramatic rescue of the submarine USS Squalus [5] in 243 feet of the Atlantic Ocean, the salvage operation provided the first real test of NEDU's helium-oxygen breathing mixture. Unfortunately, 26 of the crew drowned, while only 33 were saved. After divers experienced disorienting nitrogen narcosis while breathing air, they were switched to helium. Breathing helium eliminated the effects of nitrogen narcosis and allowed the divers to work longer and more efficiently. The low solubility of water made helium a good alternative to nitrogen in reducing the incidence of nitrogen bubble formation responsible for "decompression sickness," and "nitrogen narcosis" in underwater diving.

From the 1930s to the 1970s, there was a lack of systematic research on heliox. However, studies conducted up to the present day have examined the effects of heliox use on various outcomes. From a physiological perspective, helium reduces the effort required for breathing and enhances the gas supply to the lungs, and these effects are attributed to its physical properties. The work of breathing in patients is influenced by the compliance of the respiratory system and the resistance of the airways. Specifically, the impact of a gas on airflow through an airway and airway resistance is determined by factors such as the density and viscosity of the inspired gas, as well as the size, shape, and flow rate of the airways. A substance with higher viscosity leads to increased friction and greater breathing effort when compared to a gas with lower viscosity. The viscosity of air affects the type of airflow in the airway. Airflow can be laminar, turbulent, or transitional, which is somewhere in between the two. During inspiration and exhalation, air particles travel through the airways in a straight, laminar flow under the influence of a constant pressure gradient. When there is a partial airway obstruction, the airflow that should be laminar may become turbulent. Turbulent flow is characterized by vortices and fluctuations. This obstruction increases airway resistance, leading to an increase in the work of breathing, which can cause respiratory failure requiring orotracheal intubation and mechanical ventilation. [5]. Turbulent flow, unlike laminar flow, is impacted by the density of a gas. Therefore, a less dense gas, such as a helium-oxygen mixture, flows more efficiently under turbulent conditions and reduces the pressure needed to generate the flow. Since the pressure required to produce flow is directly proportional to the density of the gas, according to Bernoulli's principle, less pressure is needed to move the less dense gas, like heliox, through a partially obstructed airway than is needed for air or oxygen. This reduction in pressure decreases respiratory resistance and fatigue [6].

Clinical Results

Systematic research on heliox was limited until the 1970s. During that time, studies on its potential benefits in treating upper airway obstruction showed conflicting results. In recent years, research has primarily focused on pediatric populations, particularly in the treatment of both upper airway obstruction (UAO) and lower airway obstruction (LAO), such as asthma. In adults, the only randomized clinical trials have examined the use of heliox in treating asthma or COPD exacerbations. Most studies on heliox are hindered by small sample sizes. Additionally, due to the emergent nature of severe airway obstructions, controlled studies in these areas are scarce [6-7].

In 1990, Gluck and colleagues [8] studied seven mechanically ventilated adults with status asthmaticus who developed persistent respiratory acidosis associated with high airway pressures. They were treated using a 60:40 heliox mixture, resulting in a dramatic resolution of the acidosis within 20 minutes. In six of the patients, there was a significant decrease in peak inspiratory pressure (PIP) and arterial carbon dioxide (PaCO2), which helped correct respiratory acidosis within minutes of heliox administration. No adverse effects were reported. The study concludes that heliox should be considered for use in mechanically ventilated asthmatics with respiratory acidosis who fail conventional therapy. In 1995, Kass and Castriotta [9] conducted an unblinded study of 12 adults with severe asthma, suggesting a positive benefit to early treatment with heliox in adult asthmatics. The 12 patients all had acute respiratory acidosis (pH < 7.35 and PCO2 > 44 mm Hg). Before receiving heliox, all patients had been treated with 3-5 doses of nebulized albuterol. Five of the patients were on mechanical ventilation, while the other 7 received heliox through a face mask. They all received a mixture of 60% to 70% helium and 30% to 40% oxygen. After heliox administration, there was a significant decrease in PCO2 (57.9 to 47.5 mm Hg) and a significant increase in pH (7.23 to 7.32) at an average of 49.2 minutes. The researchers found that 4 of the patients did not respond to the treatment, and these patients were different from the responders in that they had a longer duration of symptoms before treatment (over 96 hours) and a higher pretreatment pH. The investigators concluded that heliox can benefit patients with severe acute asthma, respiratory acidosis, and a short duration of symptoms. In 1999, Schaeffer and colleagues [10] conducted a retrospective case-match control design to compare the changes in alveolar to arterial gradient [(A-a) gradient] in the first 2 hours of mechanical ventilation (MV) for status asthmaticus (SA) in patients who received heliox with those who did not. They studied a total of 22 adult and pediatric ICU patients with asthmatic status, all of whom required intubation. Specifically, they compared 11 patients who received heliox in the first 2 hours of MV for SA with 11 case-matched controls who did not receive heliox.

The researchers found a significant drop in the A-a gradient in the heliox group, which allowed for the weaning of FiO2 to decrease the risk of oxygen toxicity and enable a greater percentage of helium to be used. They concluded that this approach allows for the full potential of heliox to be realized in even the most severe asthmatics.

In 2000, Gross and colleagues conducted a case series in a pediatric intensive care unit at a children's hospital. They studied 10 mechanically ventilated children with bronchiolitis. The study used a non-randomized, unblinded, repeated-measures design [11]. The infants, aged 1–9 months, were mechanically ventilated in synchronized intermittent mandatory ventilation (SIMV) mode. The researchers tested different gas mixtures at 15-minute intervals: 50:50 nitrogen-oxygen, 50:50 heliox, 60:40 heliox, 70:30 heliox, and return to 50:50 nitrogen-oxygen. The study found that using helium-oxygen mixtures did not significantly improve gas exchange in these patients. Neither ventilation nor oxygenation was noticeably improved using helium-oxygen mixtures over a nitrogen-oxygen mixture. Therefore, the study concluded that the helium-oxygen mixture does not improve gas exchange in mechanically ventilated children with bronchiolitis. In 2000, Tassaux and colleagues conducted a prospective interventional study in a medical ICU, involving 23 intubated, sedated, paralyzed, and mechanically ventilated COPD patients who were enrolled within 36 hours after intubation [12]. Their study found that using heliox resulted in significant reductions in trapped lung volume, intrinsic PEEP, peak airway pressure, and mean airway pressure. However, these improvements reverted to their baseline values after heliox was discontinued. The study also found no significant differences in various cardiovascular and respiratory parameters, leading to the conclusion that heliox did not improve cardiac performance.

In 2001, Gerbeaux et al., conducted a retrospective study of 81 patients admitted for exacerbation of COPD and respiratory acidosis [13]. In this non-randomized uncontrolled clinical study, 39 patients received a 70:30 heliox mixture (70% helium and 30% oxygen), while 42 did not receive heliox. There were no significant differences in age, gender, medical history, other treatments, clinical cardiorespiratory variables, or gas exchange upon admission to the emergency department. Among those who received heliox, the intubation rate was lower (8% vs 50%, $p < 0.01$), mortality was lower (3%

vs 24%, $p < 0.01$), and intensive care unit (ICU) admissions were nonsignificantly lower (46% vs 60%, $p = 0.23$). Among the survivors, the mean ICU stay was shorter (8 vs 18 days, $p < 0.01$). Heliox therapy seems to be beneficial as a symptomatic adjunctive therapy for acute obstructive hypoventilation. In 2002, Martinon-Torres et al., conducted a prospective, interventional, comparative study on 38 intubated infants aged 1 month to 2 years old, who were consecutively admitted to the pediatric intensive care unit (PICU) with moderate to severe RSV bronchiolitis, which is the most common severe lower respiratory tract infection in infants and young children [14]. The study aimed to assess the therapeutic effects of breathing a low-density gas mixture (heliox: 70% helium and 30% oxygen). The first 19 patients received supportive care and nebulized epinephrine, while the subsequent 19 patients also received heliox via a non-rebreather face mask. The study indicated that heliox therapy improved the patients' clinical respiratory status, as evidenced by the marked improvement in their clinical scores, reduction in accompanying tachycardia and tachypnea, and a reduced duration of hospitalization in the PICU for heliox-treated patients. In 2003, Abd-Allah and colleagues conducted a retrospective review of all severely asthmatic pediatric patients who were admitted to the pediatric intensive care unit and required mechanical ventilation [15]. They identified 28 children who required mechanical ventilation, with a mean patient age of 8.8 years (range, 1.1-14.6). All of these children had status asthmaticus and received volume-controlled ventilation using a Siemens Servo 900C ventilator. Additionally, all of them received helium-oxygen therapy as part of standard treatment at the study hospital. The researchers found that after the patients received inhaled heliox, there was a significant decrease in mean peak inspiratory pressure (PIP) from 40.5 to 35.3 cm H2O. The mean pH increased significantly from 7.26 to 7.32, and the mean partial pressure of carbon dioxide (CO2) decreased significantly from 58.2 to 50.5 mm Hg, resulting in improved blood gas levels. The authors concluded that heliox is safe and may provide a clinical advantage for mechanically ventilated patients with status asthmaticus. In 2003 a Prospective, interventional study in the intensive care unit, Jolliet et al., ten intubated, sedated, paralyzed, mechanically ventilated COPD patients studied in the following conditions: (a) baseline settings made by clinician in charge, air/O(2), ZEEP; (b) He/O(2), ZEEP; (c) air/O(2), ZEEP; (d) air/O(2), PEEPe 80% of PEEPi [16]. Measurements at each condition included V(A)/Q by the multiple inert gas elimination technique (MIGET). The researchers found that in patients with COPD on mechanical ventilation, heliox reduced intrinsic PEEP, trapped gas volume, and the inspiratory and expiratory resistance of the respiratory system. Heliox did not significantly affect the ventilation-perfusion relationships.

In a study conducted in 2005, Lee and colleagues looked at 25 mechanically ventilated patients with COPD and systolic blood pressure variations greater than 15 mm Hg to see if heliox could improve their cardiac performance [17]. They measured respiratory rate, airway pressure, flow, and inspiratory/expiratory ratio directly from the ventilator. Arterial oxygen saturation was recorded using pulse oximetry. Ten patients had pulmonary artery catheters, and the researchers measured right atrial pressure, pulmonary arterial pressure, and pulmonary arterial occlusion pressure throughout the respiratory cycle and at end-expiration. They also recorded heart rate, cardiac output, and cardiac index. The study found that mean pulmonary arterial pressure, right atrial pressure, and pulmonary arterial occlusion pressure all significantly decreased when the patients were breathing heliox. Additionally, cardiac index increased by more than 20% in the heliox group. There were no significant changes in heart rate, mean arterial pressure, arterial oxygen levels, carbon dioxide levels, or pH between the control and heliox groups. Improvements were also seen in left ventricular performance, with respiratory changes in systolic pressure variations (DPP) decreasing by more than 50% during heliox breathing, and minimal pulse pressure (PPmin) increasing significantly during expiration. Furthermore, peak airway pressure, plateau pressure, intrinsic positive end-expiratory pressure (PEEPi), and trapped lung volume at end-expiration, also known as functional residual capacity (FRC), all decreased significantly during heliox ventilation. Lee concluded that heliox may be a useful additional therapy for patients with severe chronic obstructive pulmonary disease during acute respiratory failure who experience persistent intrinsic positive end-expiratory pressure-induced hemodynamic changes despite ventilator management. In 2014, Beurskens et al., conducted an observational cohort substudy [18] involving twenty-four ICU patients who were admitted after a cardiac arrest and mechanically ventilated for 3 hours with heliox (50% helium; 50% oxygen). This population was studied as part of a feasibility study investigating the neuroprotective properties of heliox [19]. A fixed protective ventilation protocol (6 mL/kg) was used, and changes in lung mechanics and gas exchange were prospectively observed. All patients were also treated with therapeutic hypothermia (32°C–34°C) as part of standard care for those with decreased consciousness after CPR. The results showed that during heliox ventilation, respiratory rate decreased (25 ± 4 versus 23 ± 5 breaths min(-1), $P = 0.010$). Minute volume ventilation showed a trend to decrease compared to baseline (11.1 ± 1.9 versus 9.9 ± 2.1 L min(-1),

$P = 0.026$), while reducing $PaCO_2$ levels (5.0 ± 0.6 versus 4.5 ± 0.6 kPa, $P = 0.011$) and peak pressures (21.1 ± 3.3 versus 19.8 ± 3.2 cm H_2O, $P = 0.024$). The researchers concluded that heliox improved CO_2 elimination while allowing reduced minute volume ventilation in adult patients during protective mechanical ventilation.

Effects of Heliox on Aerosol and Nebulization Delivery

In patients who are on mechanical ventilation and have airway obstruction, using a mixture of helium and oxygen ($He–O_2$) can help reduce airway resistance and improve ventilation. However, it's unclear how these mixtures affect the delivery of aerosols or nebulized medications. The type of gas used to power the nebulizer can impact its performance. Hess et al., [20] studied the impact of heliox (80% helium, 20% oxygen) on nebulizer function. They found that when the nebulizer was powered with heliox, the amount of albuterol inhaled was significantly reduced, and the time required for nebulization more than doubled compared to when the nebulizer was powered with air. A higher flow rate with heliox led to a similar amount of respirable medication output as with air, which can be explained by Bernoulli's principle. This principle predicts that the decreased density of heliox increases the speed at which the gas leaves the jet orifice and generates less negative pressure to draw in the drug solution. Several studies have shown that aerosols penetrate the lungs more effectively in patients with stable asthma and acute airway constriction when using heliox [21-22].

The lower density and greater viscosity of heliox result in less turbulent gas flow, which is thought to improve the transport of aerosols through narrow airways to the outer areas of the lungs. Henderson et al., found no significant advantage of heliox-driven nebulizer therapy over oxygen-driven nebulizer therapy [23]. However, they did not consider the impact of heliox on nebulizer function, which may have affected their findings negatively.

Goode et al., studied the impact of various $He-O_2$ mixtures on albuterol delivery from metered-dose inhalers (MDIs) and jet nebulizers in a simulated mechanical ventilation setting [24]. They discovered that albuterol delivery from an MDI was enhanced when the ventilator circuit contained 80% helium and 20% oxygen ($He-O_2$ 80/20) compared to other mixtures. The difference was mainly due to decreased drug deposition in the spacer chamber. Nebulizer efficiency at a flow rate of 6 L/min was five times lower with a $He-O_2$ mixture (80% helium and 20% oxygen) than with pure oxygen. The amount of nebulized drug was inversely correlated with gas density. When the nebulizer was operated with oxygen, greater albuterol delivery was achieved when the ventilator circuit contained a He-O2 mixture rather than pure oxygen.

In summary, He-O2 mixtures in the circuit increased aerosol delivery for both metered-dose inhalers (MDIs) and nebulizers in the mechanically ventilated model by as much as 50%. In conclusion, at appropriate flow rates and concentrations, He-O2 in the ventilator circuit may improve aerosol delivery in mechanically ventilated patients with severe airway obstruction [25]. In a study by Diehl et al., the effects of heliox at the end of the weaning process on work of breathing were examined [26]. The study involved a prospective randomized crossover study with 13 patients with COPD. The patients were evaluated before and after extubation. Heliox and air-oxygen were administered sequentially for 20 minutes each, in a randomized order, just before extubation. The study was repeated after extubation with five of the patients. Results showed that while heliox did not affect the breathing pattern, it reduced the work of breathing by 21%, mainly by reducing the resistive component of the work of breathing. Lower intrinsic PEEP was also found with heliox. It was observed that all patients who had an improvement in work of breathing had very high initial values. Additionally, there was a 15% reduction in respiratory rate, a 30% increase in VT (tidal volume), a 13% increase in minute ventilation, and a 29% increase in maximum inspiratory flow.

Respirator Performance with Heliox

To ensure mechanical ventilators work properly, it is essential to have accurate flow measurement for calculating delivered volume and for proper gas mixing. These functions are calibrated based on the use of nitrogen-oxygen gas mixtures, which have consistent density when mixed. However, the use of helium can significantly impact the operation of the ventilator. When administering helium during mechanical ventilation, constant monitoring and vigilance are necessary, as helium can disrupt ventilator operation and affect the accuracy of the pneumotachometer. Several studies have compared the effects of helium and various heliox mixtures on different ventilators for both adult and neonatal patients, and the results varied [27, 28]. It has been observed that the delivered tidal volume (VT) varies across different ventilator models, and the delivered fraction of inspired oxygen (FiO2) can be higher or lower than the set value. Differences have also been noted in ventilation modes, such as pressure or volume control [29]. Tassaux and colleagues have developed correction factors for ventilators with similar design characteristics. These discrepancies are specific to each ventilator and ventilation mode, so it's important to be cautious when using helium ventilation in clinical practice. The reasons for these differences are explained below. In some ventilator models (Veolar FT, Galileo, and Servo 900C), there is a single inspiratory valve downstream of the gas mixer, which is calibrated using a single FiO2 value. Because there is no integrated system to adjust to changes in gas density, the gas flow through the circuit needs to increase during volume-controlled ventilation with heliox. This effect will be more pronounced with higher concentrations of helium.

When using ventilators with high gas flow rates, the delivered tidal volume (VT) may be higher than the set VT. In some ventilator models, gas mixing happens before the inspiratory valve, meaning that oxygen delivery is not impacted by the addition of helium. However, in ventilator models equipped with two proportional inspiratory valves, gas mixing occurs after these valves, affecting the delivered VT in volume-controlled ventilation and reducing the FIO2 proportional to the helium concentration. In ventilators with leak compensation, such as the Avoid 4, the expiratory flow sensor may not function properly with heliox, leading to the sensor interpreting it as a gas leak in the circuit. This triggers an increase in the opening of the inspiratory valve, further increasing the delivered VT. On the other hand, the Servo 900C ensures consistent FIO2 delivery as gas mixing happens close to the inspiratory valve. However, the Servo 900C's scissor valve is influenced by gas density, causing the delivered VT to differ from the set VT. In the Servo 300 and Servo-i ventilators, the air and oxygen modules operate separately, each with its own supply pressure and temperature transducer. When helium is introduced into the air inlet, the increased flow leads to a larger volume in the chamber, increasing the pressure and stopping the flow, preventing the VT from being exceeded. Moreover, when pure helium is connected to the air inlet, the delivered VT is more affected than with Heliox.

Practical Aspect

When using ventilators that do not deliver a consistent FIO2, it is important to measure the FIO2 close to the patient using devices that are density-independent to ensure greater consistency. There are two practical solutions to ensure consistent VT delivery. One option is to use a conversion factor specific to each ventilator, as suggested by Tassaux et al., and estimate the delivered VT from the set VT or the exhaled VT. Alternatively, VT can be measured directly at the endotracheal tube using a density-independent pneumotachometer or one calibrated for helium. The CO2SMO pulmonary function monitor is calibrated for helium, and its measured VT with heliox is accurate, matching the volume measurements made with a volume-displacement (density-independent) spirometer (unpublished data).

Conclusion

Heliox, due to its lower density compared to air or oxygen, increases gas particle deposition and improves airflow through constricted passageways by transforming turbulent flow into laminar flow. Studies have demonstrated significant effects on patients, with benefits seen quickly, usually within an hour of treatment initiation. These effects include a reduction in respiratory rate, an increase in tidal volume, an increase in minute ventilation and maximum inspiratory flow, a mean reduction in trapped lung volume and intrinsic PEEP, lower peak and mean airway pressure, a reduction in inspiratory and expiratory resistance, and improvement in work of breathing. These effects also resulted in a drop in the A-a gradient, correction of severe respiratory acidosis, and reduction of accompanying tachycardia and tachypnea. Therefore, heliox led to a reduction in the intubation rate in patients with asthma and COPD, lower mortality, and reduced hospitalization time.

Key Messages

Based on the available evidence, the indications for using heliox during mechanical ventilation are:

1. Lower airway obstruction, especially with hypercarbia such as Asthma and COPD
2. Need to enhance aerosol delivery to lung periphery
3. Need to facilitate weaning from mechanical ventilation
4. Some ventilators perform relatively well with heliox and are not substantially affected by it. It is preferable to connect the heliox to the air inlet of the ventilator, as this results in more consistent delivery of

oxygen and tidal volume. When administering heliox, pay close attention and directly monitor the actual tidal volume and actual fraction of inspired oxygen (FiO2).

In conclusion, due to the physical properties of helium and its effects on lung function during pathological events, the helium-oxygen mixture and its clinical applications provide clinicians with an effective tool for managing respiratory emergencies.

References

[1] Slutsky, A. S. Mechanical Ventilation. *Chest* 1993; 104(6), 1833–1859.

[2] Silva, P. L., Rocco, P. R. M. The basics of respiratory mechanics: ventilator-derived parameters, Review *Ann Transl Med* 2018; Oct 1;6(19):376.

[3] Lockyer, W. J. S, Helium: Its Discovery and Applications. *Nature* 1920; May 1, 105, 360–363.

[4] Barach, AL. The therapeutic use of helium. *JAMA* 1935, October 17; 107:1273–1280.

[5] U.S. Navy. Bureau of Medicine and Surgery. *The History of the Medical Department of the United States Navy in World War II Volume* 1: A Narrative and Pictorial Volume. 1953.

[6] McGarvey, J. M., Pollack, C. J. Heliox in airway management Review *Emerg Med Clin North Am* 2008; Nov 1;26(4):905-20.

[7] Venkataraman, S. T., Heliox during mechanical ventilation. *Respir Care* 2006 Jun 1;51(6):632-9.

[8] Gluck, E., Onorato, D., Castriotta, R. Helium-oxygen mixtures in intubated patients with status asthmaticus and respiratory acidosis. *Chest* 1990, September 1; 98(3):693–698.

[9] Kass, J., Castriotta, R. Heliox therapy in acute severe asthma. *Chest* 1995 March 1; 107(3):757–760.

[10] Schaeffer, E. M., Pohlman, A., Morgan, S., Hall, J. B. Oxygenation in status asthmaticus improves during ventilation with helium-oxygen. *Crit Care Med* 1999, December 1;27(12):2666–2670.

[11] Gross, M. F., Spear, R. M., Peterson, B. M. Helium-oxygen mixture does not improve gas exchange in mechanically ventilated children with bronchiolitis, *Crit Care* 2000, Apr 13;4(3):188-92.

[12] Tassaux, D., Jolliet, P., Roeseler, J., Chevrolet, J. C. Effects of helium-oxygen on intrinsic positive end-expiratory pressure in intubated and mechanically ventilated patients with severe chronic obstructive pulmonary disease. *Crit Care Med* 2000 Aug ;28(8):2721-8.

[13] Gerbeaux, P. Gaannier, M., Boussuges, et al., Use of heliox in patients with severe exacerbation of chronic obstructive pulmonary disease. *Crit Care Med* 2001, December 1;29(12):2322–2324.

[14] Martinón-Torres, F., Rodríguez-Núñez, A., & Martinón-Sánchez, J. M. (2002, January 1) Heliox therapy in infants with acute bronchiolitis. *Pediatrics* 2002; 109:68–73.

[15] Abd-Allah, S. A., Rogers, M. S., Terry, et al., Helium oxygen therapy for pediatric acute severe asthma requiring mechanical ventilation. *Pediatr Crit Care Med* 2003, July 14(3):353–357.

[16] Jolliet, P., Watremez, C., Roeseler, J., et al., Comparative effects of helium-oxygen and external positive end-expiratory pressure on respiratory mechanics, gas exchange, and ventilation-perfusion relationships in mechanically ventilated patients with chronic obstructive pulmonary disease. *Intensive Care Med* 2003, July 8, 9;29,9,1442–1450.

[17] Lee, D. L., Lee, H., Wen Chang, H., et al., Heliox improves hemodynamics in mechanically ventilated patients with chronic obstructive pulmonary disease with systolic pressure variations. *Crit Care Med* 2005, May 1;33(5):968-73.

[18] Beurskens, C. J., Brevoord, D., Lagrand, W. K., et al., Heliox Improves Carbon Dioxide Removal during Lung Protective Mechanical Ventilation. *Crit Care Res Pract* 2014, January 1:2014:954814.

[19] Brevoord D., Beurskens C., Juffermans N., et al., Helium ventilation is safe and feasible in ICU patients admitted after cardiac arrest. *Critical Care* 2012, March 20.

[20] Hess, D. R., Acosta F. L., Ritz R. H., The effect of heliox on nebulizer function using a β-agonist bronchodilator. *Chest* 1999, January 1;115(1):184–189.

[21] Svartengren, M., Anderson, M., Philipson, K., Camner, P. Human lung deposition of particles suspended in air or in helium/oxygen mixture. *Exp Lung Res* 1989, January 1;15(4):575–585.

[22] Anderson, M., Svartengren, M., Bylin, G., et al., Deposition in asthmatics of particles inhaled in air or in helium-oxygen. *Am Rev Respir Dis* 1993, march 1;147(3):524–52.

[23] Henderson, S. O., Acharya, P., Kilaghbian, T., et al., Use of heliox-driven nebulizer therapy in the treatment of acute asthma. *Ann Emerg Med* 1999, February 1;33(2):141–146.

[24] Goode, M. L., Fink, J. B., Dhand, R., Tobin, M. J. Improvement in aerosol delivery with helium-oxygen mixtures during mechanical ventilation. *Am J Respir Crit Care Med* 2001;163(1):109–114.

[25] Hess, D. R., Fink, J. B., Venkataraman, S. T., et al., The history and physics of heliox. *Respir Care* 2006;51(6):608–12.

[26] Diehl, J. L., Mercat, A., Guerot, E., et al., Helium/oxygen mixture reduces the work of breathing at the end of the weaning process in patients with severe chronic obstructive pulmonary disease. *Crit Care Med* 2003;31(5): 1415–1420.

[27] Tassaux, D., Jolliet, P., Thouret, J. M., et al., Calibration of seven ICU ventilators for mechanical ventilation with helium-oxygen mixtures. *Am J Respir Crit Care Med* 1999;160(1): 22–32.

[28] Oppenheim, E. A., Cohen, Y., Weissman, C., Pizov, R. The effect of helium on ventilator performance: study of five ventilators and a bedside Pitot tube spirometer. *Chest* 2001;120(2):582–588.

[29] Berkenbosch, J. W., Grueber, R. E., Dabbagh, O., McKibben, A. W. Effect of helium-oxygen (heliox) gas mixtures on the function of four pediatric ventilators. *Crit Care Med* 2003 ;31(7):2052–2058.

Chapter 16

Heliox Therapy and Weaning from Mechanical Ventilation

Maria Barbagallo*, MD
and Eleonora Schiappa, MD
Department of Anesthesiology and Critical Care, University Hospital of Parma, Parma, OH, USA

Abstract

For some patients, weaning from ventilation is a challenge. Difficult weaning represents a clinical problem because morbidity and even mortality may be higher. In some cases, heliox could serve as an effective additional therapy, allowing for clinical improvement and providing time for standard therapy to work. Helium is an inert gas with a lower density than air; thus, its flow through an airway is less turbulent, leading to lower resistance. Inhalation of heliox, instead of air, significantly reduces airway resistance. Helium could facilitate the period after extubation in selected patients who develop respiratory distress shortly after extubation and may help avoid reintubation. It offers potential benefits for newborn infants affected by respiratory distress syndrome (RDS). In intubated chronic obstructive pulmonary disease (COPD), it enhances lung emptying, decreases PEEPi, and improves patient-ventilator interaction and tolerance to spontaneous-assisted breathing, which, in turn, may facilitate weaning and lead to better patient outcomes.

Keywords: extubation, heliox ventilation, mechanical ventilation, post-extubation stridor, weaning

* Corresponding Author's Email: mbarbagallo@ao.pr.it

In: Respiratory Care in Heliox Therapy Physiology and Technology
Editor: Antonio M. Esquinas
ISBN: 979-8-89530-385-6

Introduction

Weaning from mechanical ventilation represents the period of transition from total ventilatory support to spontaneous breathing and consists in a gradual decrease in ventilatory support [1, 2]. Recovering PaO_2/FiO_2 ratios, lower FiO_2 requirements and lower ventilator settings might indicate the initiation of weaning readiness assessment. Weaning success is defined as extubation and the absence of ventilatory support 48 hours after extubation. Conversely, weaning failure is defined as the inability to pass a spontaneous breathing trial (SBT) or the need for reintubation within 48 hour a following extubation [1].

Patients who are difficult to wean represent a clinical challenge as they usually require a longer hospital stay and have higher morbidity and mortality rates. It has been reported that the weaning period accounts for 40% of the total duration of mechanical ventilatory support, so every effort should be made to determine, as soon as possible, which patients can be rapidly extubated, while minimizing the weaning period [1].

The first step is to recognize when a patient is ready to be weaned. A daily follow-up routine should be performed for every intubated, mechanically ventilated patient. Sedation vacations play a major role in readiness assessments. Reversible contributors to respiratory failure (e.g., electrolyte imbalances, volume overload, pneumonia, and other pathophysiologic factors) should be corrected. Subsequently, objective criteria to further assess readiness should be applied [1]. Classically, when patients meet these criteria, they are allowed to breathe spontaneously for a period that may range from several minutes to several hours before the decision to extubate is made.

Weaning failure may depend on several factors and is often due to more than one cause. The main reasons for weaning failure include abnormal gas exchange, cardiovascular instability, psychological dependence on the ventilator, and respiratory pump failure [1]. Additionally, malnutrition, cognitive, diaphragmatic, metabolic, endocrine, gastro-intestinal, and renal dysfunctions are also contributing factors to weaning failure [1].

Regardless of the underlying disorder that necessitates mechanical ventilation (MV), the most common mechanism is generally an imbalance between the force-generating capacity of the respiratory muscles and the load they must face once MV is discontinued.

Since Barach (1934) first described heliox (He/O_2), a mixture of helium and oxygen, as an effective treatment for diseases involving airway obstruction, numerous studies have been conducted in both animals and humans examining its effectiveness [2]. Studies from the 1930s to the present have measured the impact of heliox use on a variety of outcomes, including peak flow, dyspnea scores, arterial blood gas values, peak airway pressures, exercise performance and pulmonary function test variables. It has been shown to be a useful adjunctive therapy in children with asthma, bronchiolitis, upper airway obstruction, acute respiratory distress, post-extubation stridor [2].

Helium is an inert gas with a lower density than air, thus allowing the flow of helium through an airway to be less turbulent, leading to lower resistance [2]. Inhalation of heliox, instead of air, significantly reduces airway resistance, and during He/O_2 ventilation, lower driving pressures are necessary to distribute oxygen to the distal alveoli, thereby improving oxygenation [3].

Breathing heliox decreases air-trapping in (and hyperinflation of) the lungs (caused by lower-airway obstruction), thereby reducing intrinsic positive end-expiratory pressure (PEEPi) [4]. Heliox decreases dyspnea and work of breathing, and improves distal-airway deposition of aerosol particles [4]. Heliox ventilation is associated with a higher expiratory flow when compared to standard mixtures at the same pressure. This may facilitate passive exhalation, offsetting the danger of gas trapping and the accompanying barotrauma. Several studies reported a decrease in the oxygen demand with heliox ventilation [4].

It has been reported that heliox ventilation reduces respiratory effort, diaphragmatic load and displays protective effects against atelectasis and airway collapse [4]. Also, diffusion capacities of CO_2 are increased, further improving gas exchange [2]. Another potential benefit of helium is its possible anti-inflammatory properties [4]. Helium-oxygen ventilation has been reported to result in a significant decrease of serum inflammatory markers such as IL-6, IL-8, CRP, and TNFα in neonates with meconium aspiration, with similar findings observed in animal models [4].

Recent Findings. Potential Uses of Heliox in Weaning

Chronic Obstructive Pulmonary Disease (COPD)

Patients with COPD who require mechanical ventilation generally have a significant dependence on ventilators [5]. Reports from two specialized weaning units indicate that only 22% to 35% of patients with COPD can eventually be liberated from the ventilator, and 19% of those remain partially dependent on the ventilator [5].

Weaning COPD patients from mechanical ventilation is a particularly difficult issue. The reasons for this are primarily related to respiratory muscle weakness, abnormalities in arterial blood gases, malnutrition, disturbances in respiratory system mechanics, and eventually other co-morbidities, such as renal failure or coronary artery disease [5].

For decompensated COPD-patients, there is a marked increase in both the elastic and resistive components of the work of breathing (WOB) [6]. The resulting respiratory muscle fatigue is a key factor in determining weaning trial failure and prolonged ventilator dependence in intubated patients [6]. Moreover, pulmonary inflation decreases the inspiratory contractile capacity by putting the respiratory muscles in an unfavorable position on their tension-length curves [7].

Considerable literature exists describing modalities that assist in weaning COPD patients from invasive ventilation. Pressure support (PS) is often used to provide a titratable level of respiratory muscle unloading in these patients [7]. However, excessive levels of PS can adversely affect patient-ventilator synchrony and increase WOB [7]. Likewise, applying external positive end-expiratory pressure (PEEPe) can counteract the inspiratory threshold effect of intrinsic PEEP (PEEPi), but PEEPe may be difficult to titrate and can increase total PEEP and dynamic hyperinflation [6].

Several studies have speculated on the potential use of heliox during the weaning process for COPD patients. Lowering the density of the inspiratory gas mixture, using heliox could provide two main benefits [7]. First, it could facilitate the transition from turbulent to laminar flows by lowering the Reynolds number, and second, it could reduce driving pressure in areas where flow remains turbulent, as well as in other areas where flow patterns are transitional due to the complex geometry of the airway tree. Both effects are expected to reduce driving pressure, thus unloading the respiratory system. Conversely, the higher viscosity of the helium/oxygen mixture, compared to the air/oxygen mixture could exert a contrary effect in areas of laminar flows. Indeed, in such areas, Poisseuille's law indicates that for a given flow, the pressure decrease is proportional to the viscosity. The low density of helium compared to air can decrease resistances to gas flow and work of breathing in patients with airflow limitation [7].

Tassaux et al., demonstrated that in intubated patients with severe COPD ventilated with pressure support, He/O_2 decreases the level of PEEPi and the number of ineffective inspiratory attempts. It also reduces the magnitude of inspiratory efforts and the total WOB as well as its resistive and elastic components [6]. A decrease in dynamic hyperinflation has also been shown [6].

Gainnier et al., obtained similar results in patients undergoing controlled ventilation, documenting a reduction in total, resistive, and elastic WOB with He/O_2 [8].

Diehl et al., choose to study the effects of the mixture in spontaneously breathing COPD patients recovering from an acute exacerbation. They conducted a prospective randomized crossover study involving 13 COPD patients, evaluated in a stable condition just before and after extubation [7]. Heliox and air-oxygen were administered sequentially, for 20 minutes each in a randomized order, just before extubation. They demonstrated that the helium/oxygen mixture can lower the work of breathing and dynamic hyperinflation in COPD patients at the end of the weaning process, without affecting the breathing pattern. Partial data also suggested that these beneficial effects can be observed after extubation [7]. In the whole group studied before extubation, they found a 21% reduction in the WOB, consistent with data previously reported by Jaber and colleagues [9]. These authors studied the combined effects of the helium/oxygen mixture with noninvasive ventilation (NIV) in ten COPD patients with acute exacerbation. Nine of these patients were studied on low-pressure support, mimicking spontaneous breathing. In this condition, the helium/oxygen mixture induced a similar mean reduction of 21% in the WOB [9].

Jolliet et al., found that noninvasive positive-pressure support ventilation with heliox decreased $PaCO_2$ and dyspnea in decompensated COPD patients [10].

Lin Lee et al., recruited 25 mechanically ventilated patients with COPD suffering from acute respiratory failure who having a systolic pressure variation of 15 mm Hg [3]. Heliox ventilation was applied as an adjunct therapy within 24 hours of mechanical ventilation. Ventilation with heliox may facilitate lung emptying, reduce PEEPi, and improve hemodynamics. They also observed improvement in cardiac performance, as shown by a reduction in pulse pressure (PP) and increases in the cardiac index. The reduction in PP with heliox likely reflected the attenuation of PEEPi-induced depression of cardiac output with concomitant increase in venous return [3].

Post-Extubation Stridor (PES)

Endotracheal intubation can lead to inflammation and swelling around the airway, resulting in upper and total airway resistance, which may cause increased inspiratory effort [11]. Approximately 5% to 16% of patients develop post-extubation airway obstruction and respiratory distress [11]. In addition, many patients develop inspiratory distress after extubation, leading to reintubation [11]. In these patients, an increase in upper airway and total inspiratory resistance can contribute to this respiratory distress. Some studies showed that helium-oxygen (He/O_2) therapy can provide beneficial effects for upper airway obstruction during the post-extubation period, reducing the effort required for breathing [11].

Jaber et al., evaluated the effects of a helium-oxygen mixture on inspiratory effort, blood gases, and comfort in non-COPD patients intubated for at least 48 hours [11]. They found that using He/O_2 instead of N_2O_2 reduced inspiratory effort and improved comfort post-extubation [11].

Similarly, Skrinskas et al., reported positive outcomes using He/O_2 in 10 patients with acute upper airway obstruction [12]. Four patients developed respiratory distress after removal of an endotracheal tube, three patients had an obstruction related to radiation therapy, and three patients had a primary tumor. With the exception of one case of intermittent complete airway obstruction, the use of He/O_2 improved patients, by avoiding intubation and/or allowing time to prepare the patients for surgery [12].

In a double-blind, randomized, controlled, crossover study by Kemper et al., 13 children with burns and other trauma experienced a 38% reduction in respiratory distress scores when breathing He/O_2 compared to N_2O_2 for post-extubation stridor [13].

Pediatrics

Extremely preterm infants are frequently affected by respiratory distress syndrome (RDS) and often require mechanical ventilation. Early weaning from mechanical ventilation is desirable, but extubation failure can be prevented in several ways, including caffeine administration and use of non-invasive respiratory support, such as nasal continuous positive airway pressure (NCPAP), bi-level NCPAP (BiPAP), or nasal intermittent positive pressure ventilation (NIPPV) [14]. Despite these strategies, 25–40% of low birth weight infants and 60% of 24–26 weeks gestation infants experience extubation failure and require reinstitution of mechanical ventilation, which is associated with increased pulmonary morbidity, such as subglottic stenosis, pneumonia, ventilator-induced lung injury, and increased risk of bronchopulmonary dysplasia (BPD) [14]. Helium has been reported to be beneficial in several pediatric pathologies. Studies show that heliox can effectively decrease the resistive work of breathing in patients with RDS and enhance the efficacy of non-invasive ventilation methods, potentially reducing the need for mechanical ventilation [14].

Dani et al., evaluated the efficacy of a 24 hour course of non-invasive ventilation with heliox (Hx-NCPAP/ Hx-BiPAP) in decreasing the incidence of extubation failure in preterm infants with RDS compared with non-invasive ventilation with air-oxygen (NCPAP/BiPAP) [14]. They found that treatment with heliox non-invasive ventilation did not reduce the incidence of extubation failure in preterm infants with RDS but improved their respiratory function without adverse effects. Infants in the heliox group showed a significant decrease in $PaCO_2$ [14].

Migliori et al., performed an uncontrolled and non-blinded study to evaluate the effects of heliox on a population of preterm, long-term mechanically ventilated infants by measuring pulmonary mechanics, ventilatory parameters, and gas exchange before, during, and one hour after treatment [15]. Afterward, the infants who manifested a significant reduction of peak inspiratory pressure (PIP), while on a fixed tidal volume (TV) delivered by the ventilator, were extubated [15]. Subsequently nasal bilevel positive airway pressure (BiPAP) and heliox were administered for the following 3 hours, followed by a medical air/oxygen mixture. Gas exchange and the need for reintubation were evaluated over the next 24 hours. Heliox was well tolerated by all the patients, and none of the patients had any adverse effects [15]. Eight infants were extubated and ventilated with BiPAP and heliox for 3 hours. Only 1 of them required reintubation over the next 24 hours, 5 hours after returning to the conventional air/oxygen mixture. Their results suggest that heliox reduces WOB and the need for pressure support and improves gas exchange in preterm mechanically ventilated infants [15].

Duration of Therapy

The optimal timing and duration of He/O_2 administration remains to be determined [6]. The therapeutic effects of heliox are typically observed quickly, often within minutes of initiation. However, these effects dissipate soon after discontinuation, some authors to suggest heliox as a "therapeutic bridge" until the underlying causes of respiratory failure are resolved [4]. Thus, the clinician quickly understands if heliox therapy will be beneficial for an individual patient or whether it should be abandoned for other possible therapies [2].

Conclusion

In the ICU, it is critical to evaluate patient readiness for weaning as early as possible and to mitigate risk factors for weaning failure. For patients who fail weaning trials, a detailed structured approach to identify potential causes and mechanisms is essential. In the era of patient-customized care, it is important to select a patient-specific weaning modality.

In some cases, He/O_2 may be an interesting adjunctive therapy, allowing clinical improvement and allowing time for the usual therapy to work. Helium is an inert gas, almost insoluble in tissues and non-reactive with biologic membranes and not associated with any toxic effects. Heliox could ease the post-extubation period in selected patients who develop respiratory distress shortly after extubation and in some cases may avoid reintubation.

Heliox is beneficial for newborns due to its respiratory effects and potential cardio/neuro-protective properties, aiding in the prevention of NIV failure and reducing the risk of lung injury in pediatric patients.

In intubated COPD patients it enhances lung emptying, decreases PEEPi and the number of ineffective inspiratory attempts, and reduces the key determinants of elevated WOB and inspiratory effort. He/O_2 may therefore prove useful in patients with high levels of PEEPi and WOB by unloading the respiratory muscles. This can improve patient-ventilator interaction and tolerance to spontaneous-assisted breathing, which may in turn benefit patient outcomes by facilitating weaning.

Heliox may also be a useful adjunct therapy for improving cardiac performance in severe COPD patients who experience hemodynamic changes associated with PEEPi, despite adjustments to ventilator settings.

The optimal duration of therapy remains unknown, but it seems obvious that the length of the Heliox ventilation must be tailored to the individual needs of each patient. Future studies should aim to identify criteria for the safe weaning among other issues.

One final consideration is that despite its unique properties, heliox has not gained widespread popularity. Certain barriers seem to limit its use, including technical issues and the need for specialized equipment. Moreover, helium-oxygen mixtures are not available on demand in every country and may require special supply chains. Additionally, heliox is only provided in cylinders, and continuous wall supply is uncommon. Finally, Heliox is more expensive than oxygen or room air. Given the technical pitfalls and cost issues associated with the use of He/O_2, studies are needed to determine whether the beneficial pathophysiological effects of He/O_2 inhalation during weaning can have an impact on the duration of weaning, ICU stay, and overall patient outcomes, possibly resulting in its increased use.

Key Message

1. Patients who are difficult to wean require longer hospital stays and may experience higher morbidity and mortality
2. Helium is an inert, non-toxic gas, insoluble in tissues and nonreactive with biologic membranes that may serve as an effective adjunct therapy
3. Heliox has proven to be effective in improving patient-ventilator interaction and can facilitate weaning.
4. Heliox may benefit newborns, particularly in preventing reintubation following extubation distress.
5. The effects of heliox are relatively rapid, typically evident within minutes after initiation. The optimal duration of therapy remains unknown but must be tailored to the individual needs of each patient.

References

[1] Akella, P., L. P. Voigt, and S. Chawla. To Wean or Not to Wean: A Practical Patient Focused Guide to Ventilator Weaning. *J Intensive Care Med* 2022. 37(11): p. 1417-1425.

[2] Liet, J. M., Ducruet, T., Gupta, V., Cambonie, G Heliox inhalation therapy for bronchiolitis in infants. *Cochrane Database Syst Rev* 2015. 2015(9): p. CD006915.

[3] Lee, D. L., Lee, H., Chang, H. W., Chang, A. Y., Lin, S. L., Huang, Y. C. Heliox improves hemodynamics in mechanically ventilated patients with chronic obstructive pulmonary disease with systolic pressure variations. *Crit Care Med* 2005. 33(5): p. 968-73.

[4] Szczapa, T., P. Kwapien, and T. A. Merritt. Neonatal Applications of Heliox: A Practical Review. *Front Pediatr* 2022. 10: p. 855050.

[5] Peigang, Y. and J. J. Marini. Ventilation of patients with asthma and chronic obstructive pulmonary disease. *Curr Opin Crit Care* 2002. 8(1): p. 70-6.

[6] Tassaux, D., Gainnier, M., Battisti, A., Jolliet, P. Helium-oxygen decreases inspiratory effort and work of breathing during pressure support in intubated patients with chronic obstructive pulmonary disease. *Intensive Care Med* 2005. 31(11): p. 1501-7.

[7] Diehl, J. L., Mercat, A., Guérot, E., Aïssa, F., Teboul, J. L., Richard, C., Labrousse, J. Helium/oxygen mixture reduces the work of breathing at the end of the weaning process in patients with severe chronic obstructive pulmonary disease. *Crit Care Med* 2003. 31(5): p. 1415-20.

[8] Gainnier, M., Arnal, J. M., Gerbeaux, P., Donati, S., Papazian, L., Sainty, J. M. Helium-oxygen reduces work of breathing in mechanically ventilated patients with chronic obstructive pulmonary disease. *Intensive Care Med* 2003 29(10): p. 1666-70.

[9] Jaber, S., Fodil, R., Carlucci, A., Boussarsar, M., Pigeot, J., Lemaire, F., Harf, A., Lofaso, F., Isabey, D., and Brochard, Laurent. Noninvasive ventilation with helium-oxygen in acute exacerbations of chronic obstructive pulmonary disease. *Am J Respir Crit Care Med* 2000. 161(4 Pt 1): p. 1191-200.

[10] Jolliet, P., Tassaux, D., Roeseler, J., Burdet, L., Broccard, A., D'Hoore, W., Borst, F., Reynaert, M., Schaller, M. D., Chevrolet, J. C. Helium-oxygen versus air-oxygen noninvasive pressure support in decompensated chronic obstructive disease: A prospective, multicenter study. *Crit Care Med* 2003. 31(3): p. 878-84.

[11] Jaber, S., Carlucci, A., Boussarsar, M., Fodil, R., Pigeot, J., Maggiore, S., Harf, A., Isabey, D., Brochard, L. Helium-oxygen in the postextubation period decreases inspiratory effort. *Am J Respir Crit Care Med* 2001. 164(4): p. 633-7.

[12] Skrinskas, G. J., Hyland, R. H. and Hutcheon M. A. Using helium-oxygen mixtures in the management of acute upper airway obstruction. *Can Med Assoc J* 1983. 128(5): p. 555-8.

[13] Kemper, K. J., Izenberg, S., Marvin, J. A., Heimbach, D. M. Treatment of postextubation stridor in a pediatric patient with burns: the role of heliox. *J Burn Care Rehabil* 1990. 11(4): p. 337-9.

[14] Dani, C., Fontanelli, G., Lori, I., Favelli, F., & Poggi, C. Heliox non-invasive ventilation for preventing extubation failure in preterm infants. *J Matern Fetal Neonatal Med* 2013. 26(6): p. 603-7.

[15] Migliori, C., Gancia, P., Garzoli, E., Spinoni, V., Chirico, G. The Effects of helium/oxygen mixture (heliox) before and after extubation in long-term mechanically ventilated very low birth weight infants. *Pediatrics* 2009. 123(6): p. 1524-8.

Chapter 17

Weaning from Mechanical Ventilation Using Heliox Therapy

Mostafa Elshazly*, **MD**
and Reham Hassan Kandeel, MD
Faculty of Medicine, Cairo University, Giza, Egypt

Abstract

Mechanical ventilation (MV) weaning can be described as the process of suddenly or periodically removing ventilator support, with the primary challenge being to determine whether a patient is ready to resume spontaneous ventilation. The process begins with an assessment of readiness and ends with liberation, usually by extubation. A successful weaning process should distinguish patients who may fail extubation and require reintubation from those who are likely to succeed in maintaining spontaneous breathing without mechanical support. This is important because extubation failure and reintubation can worsen prognosis and increase the risk of mortality, length of stay, duration of mechanical ventilation, and ventilation-related complications. To guarantee a successful weaning, helium-oxygen (HeO_2) mixtures have been tested in the post-extubation period to see if such mixtures can reduce the work of breathing and improve comfort at the end of the weaning process.

Keywords: heliox, work of breathing, aerosol delivery, mechanical ventilation, weaning

* Corresponding Author's Email: melshazly@kasralainy.edu.eg

In: Respiratory Care in Heliox Therapy Physiology and Technology
Editor: Antonio M. Esquinas
ISBN: 979-8-89530-385-6

Introduction

Weaning from mechanical ventilation is defined as the process of abruptly or gradually withdrawing ventilatory support. Weaning can be considered once the underlying causes necessitating mechanical ventilation have been resolved. The process begins with a readiness assessment and ends with liberation, usually by extubations.

Liberation or weaning from mechanical ventilation is an important process that can account for 40–60% of the total duration of mechanical ventilation, making the determination of the right time to start weaning a difficult challenge [1, 2].

Two large multicenter studies have shown that mechanical ventilation can be discontinued abruptly in approximately 75% of mechanically ventilated patients whose underlying cause of respiratory failure has improved or been resolved [3]. The remaining patients will require a gradual withdrawal from mechanical ventilation.

A successful weaning process should differentiate patients who may fail extubation and need reintubation from those who are likely to succeed in maintaining spontaneous breathing without mechanical support. This is important, as extubation failure and reintubation can worsen prognosis and increase the risk of mortality, length of stay, duration of ventilation, and ventilation-related complications [4].

In 2005, following the International Consensus Conference (ICC), the process of weaning was categorized, according to expert opinion, into three groups based on the number, timing, and success of spontaneous breathing trials (SBT): simple, difficult, and prolonged weaning [5].

1. Simple weaning: Patients who are successfully weaned and extubated on the first attempt without difficulty.
2. Difficult weaning: Patients who fail initial weaning and need up to three SBTs or need up to 7 days from the first SBT to achieve successful weaning.
3. Prolonged weaning: Patients who fail at least three spontaneous breathing trials or requires more than 7 days of weaning after the first spontaneous breathing trial [6].

Weaning Criteria

Patients underwent a six-component daily screening process, which includes:

- $PaO_2/FiO_2 \geq 150$
- PEEP ≤ 5 cmH_2O
- hemodynamic stability,
- mental status
- adequate coughdd
- and f/V_T.

Patients who pass this screening automatically undergo a 2-hour SBT and are considered for extubation if the SBT is tolerated [6, 7].

Required criteria.

- PaO2/FiO2 ≥ 120–150 or SaO2 ≥ 88–90% on FiO2 ≤ 40–50% and positive end-expiratory pressure (PEEP) ≤ 5–8 cmH2O
- Hemodynamic stability (no or low doses vasopressor medications)

Additional (optional) criteria

- Weaning parameters: respiratory rate ≤35 breaths/min, spontaneous tidal volume >5 ml/kg, negative inspiratory force <−20 to −25 cmH2O, rapid shallow breathing index< 105 breaths/L/min
- Hemoglobin ≥ 8–10 mg/Dl
- Core temperature ≤ 38–38.5°C
- Mental status: awake and alert or easily arousable [6, 7].

Weaning Indices

Multiple criteria have been used to assess readiness to wean.

- Subjective criteria include tachypnoea, diaphoresis, hemodynamic stability, delirium, and other signs of increased work of breathing.
- Integrated indices include compliance, resistance, oxygenation, and pressure index; the simplified weaning index; and the rapid shallow breathing index (RSBI) [5].

Methods of weaning:

The process of discontinuing mechanical ventilation consists of four steps:

1. Stop sedation.
2. Decide whether the patient is ready to begin the weaning process.
3. Perform a spontaneous breathing trial.
4. Decide whether the patient can be extubated.

Once objective criteria for liberation are met, a spontaneous breathing trial should be conducted for patients deemed ready to wean. The SBT simulates a post-extubation state, helping to determine if the patient can adequately meet ventilator and gas exchange requirements without mechanical assistance. Formal readiness testing is conducted using a SBT with low levels of pressure support ventilation (PSV $\leq$ 7 mmHg), continuous positive airway pressure (CPAP), or unassisted through a T-piece. SBTs usually last between 30 minutes and 2 hours. Tolerance for 120 minutes of spontaneous breathing indicates that a patient no longer needs ventilatory support [3, 4].

Automated weaning modes, such as adaptive support ventilation (ASV), Smart Care/PS, proportional assist ventilation (PAV), mandatory minute ventilation, and volume support have emerged with the promise of faster weaning. Weaning from mechanical ventilation (MV) using PAV or SmartCare is associated with higher success rates compared to other methods. A total of 39 RCTs involving 5,953 patients met inclusion criteria, revealing that SmartCare and PAV were the most effective methods for increasing the success of weaning. Furthermore, PAV was superior in reducing the percentage of patients who needed reintubation and in reducing mortality rates [8].

Weaning Failure

If a patient fails an SBT, it is important to identify and correct the underlying cause prior to the next SBT. In most studies, weaning failure is defined as either the failure of the SBT or the need for reintubation within 48 hours following extubation [9]. The causes of weaning failure are categorized by physiological systems, i.e., respiratory, cardiovascular, neurological, neuropsychological, metabolic, nutritional causes (malnutrition or overweight) and anemia [9].

- Respiratory causes: hypoxemia, V/Q mismatch, dynamic hyperinflation, increased secretions, atelectasis, pleural effusion, pneumothorax.
- Cardiovascular causes: CHF deterioration, fluid overload.
- Neurological causes: decreased respiratory drive, oversedation, delirium, anxiety, depression.
- Muscular causes: respiratory muscle weakness, electrolyte disorders (hypophosphatemia, hypomagnesemia, hypocalcemia, hypokalemia), myopathy, malnutrition, hypothyroidism, hypoadrenalism, corticosteroids overuse.

A careful patient examination—including history review, physical examination, ventilator graph analysis, basic laboratory tests, and imaging studies—can often reveal the underlying cause and aid in treatment.

Once the cause of the previous SBT failure is addressed, the patient can undergo another SBT, typically lasting longer than the previous attempt (approximately 2 hours). However, if CHF is suspected as the cause for the SBT failure, it may be beneficial to perform the SBT using a T-piece to assess the patient's tolerance to the absence of PEEP.

If the patient successfully passes the SBT, extubation should be performed. However, if the patient fails, the SBT should be halted at the first signs of failure to minimize respiratory muscle fatigue.

Patients who are not able to pass an SBT after three consecutive attempts or who take more than a week to pass are considered to be undergoing prolonged weaning. Although this group represents a minority (about 10%), these patients are at increased risk of death and are more likely to need a tracheostomy [5, 6].

The Use of Heliox (Heluim/Oxygen Mixture) Therapy in Weaning Trial

Helium is an odorless, tasteless, and non-toxic gas that is noncarcinogenic and has no lasting effects on human organs. It comprises only five parts per million (0.0005%,) in the lower atmosphere. Due to its lower molecular weight and density compared to nitrogen and oxygen mixtures, it has been used to treat various respiratory-related illnesses [10].

Inhalation of heliox results in significantly lower turbulence, especially in the more distal portions of the lung. This effect translates to a greater proportion of laminar flow and lower overall airway resistance, resulting in increased flow rates by up to 50% during heliox inhalation, particularly in obstructive lung disease where airflow is restricted [11]. Therefore, heliox serves as an emergency airway solution to reduce airway resistance and respiratory muscle workload until definitive therapies can address the underlying causes in patients with asthma, chronic obstructive pulmonary disease (COPD), bronchiolitis, bronchopulmonary dysplasia and upper airway obstruction [12]. When used as a carrier, heliox has been found to improve the deposition of aerosolized bronchodilators in the lungs. The percentage of oxygen in heliox should be at least 20% to prevent hypoxia and no more than 40% to exhibit clinically significant effects. Nevertheless, the usefulness of heliox in the intensive care unit is still debatable [13].

Weaning by Heliox Therapy

Breathing a helium-oxygen mixture (HeO_2) has been investigated to determine whether it reduces inspiratory effort post-extubation. After endotracheal extubation, airway resistances may increase, resulting in high inspiratory effort and respiratory distress in 5 to 16% of patients, which can necessitate reintubation [14].

The helium-oxygen (HeO_2) mixture's low density and high kinematic viscosity allow it to reduce airway resistance, alleviating dyspnea and improving gas exchange, particularly in non-intubated patients with severe exacerbation of chronic obstructive lung disease (COPD) or asthma [12]. Recent studies have shown that helium-oxygen breathing can improve pH, $PaCO_2$ and inspiratory effort in patients with acute exacerbation of COPD, especially when combined with noninvasive pressure support ventilation [15].

In addition, the use of helium-oxygen mixtures can lower the work of breathing and the dynamic hyperinflation in COPD patients at the end of the weaning process without affecting the breathing pattern, thus unloading the respiratory system by decreasing the inspiratory resistances and dynamic hyperinflation through its effects on expiratory resistances. [16].

Abnormalities of the upper airway, including the glottis, may contribute to increased inspiratory mechanical loads following extubation, leading to post-extubation respiratory distress. Investigators have suggested a role of the supraglottic airway in explaining the increased work of breathing observed after extubation. The use of HeO_2 can reduce inspiratory effort and improve comfort after tracheal extubation. Although evidence primarily comes from observational studies, the immediate improvements obtained with HeO_2 breathing were reversed upon discontinuation, indicating a beneficial effect linked to the physical properties of the gas.

The reduced density (ρ) of HeO2, along with the negligible increase in the dynamic viscosity (μ) compared with air ($\leqslant 10\%$), results in increased kinematic viscosity ν (= μ/ρ) and a decrease in the Reynolds number (Re) leading to less turbulence and more laminar flow, thereby lowering airway resistance. These improvements lead to a decrease in inspiratory effort.

In some cases, HeO_2 may serve as an adjunctive therapy, allowing for clinical improvement and providing time for conventional treatments, such as epinephrine inhalation and corticosteroids, to take effect.

In weaning using CPAP, it is postulated that helium may act as a carrier gas for oxygen, helping to raise intra-alveolar oxygen concentration. He-CPAP offers dual advantages: it prevents or relieves atelectasis, while helium helps alleviate respiratory workload and improve oxygen diffusion into the alveoli. Consequently, the combination of the helium-oxygen mixture with continuous positive airway pressure (He-CPAP) has been employed in weaning, resulting in significant increases in PaO_2 and marked improvements in respiratory distress [17].

Although data on helium-oxygen use during weaning are limited, one physiological study aimed to determine whether breathing a helium-oxygen mixture, compared with an air-oxygen mixture during the weaning phase of mechanical ventilation, would reduce carbon dioxide production in patients without significant airways obstruction [14]. The study found that helium-oxygen significantly decreased VCO_2 production at the end of a 2-hour period of CPAP ventilation without changes in respiratory or cardiovascular parameters from their baseline's values.

Also, He/O_2 mixtures have been shown to decrease levels of PEEPi and the number of ineffective inspiratory attempts in intubated patients with severe COPD ventilated in pressure support mode, thus reducing the magnitude of inspiratory efforts and the total work of breathing, including both resistive and elastic components. Similar effects are seen in spontaneously breathing COPD patients prior to extubation, where He/O_2 reduces the level of PEEPi and the work of breathing, particularly its resistive component. In decompensated patients ventilated with noninvasive PSV via face mask, He/O_2 leads to a reduction in work of breathing [16], PaCO2, and dyspnea.

He/O_2 can also increase expiratory flow, leading to enhanced lung emptying and a decreased PEEPi by reducing expiratory airway resistance. This results in several beneficial effects: a decreased inspiratory threshold load reduces the number of non-triggering breaths and the magnitudes of esophageal pressure swings and pressure-time product (PTP). Furthermore, there is a decrease in both elastic and resistive work of breathing due to reduced PEEPi and airway resistance (Raw), suggesting that He/O2 may be particularly useful for patients with COPD who are difficult to wean [18].

He/O_2 may prove useful in patients with high levels of PEEPi and work of breathing by unloading the respiratory muscles, improving patient-ventilator synchrony and tolerance to spontaneous-assisted breathing, which in turn may be beneficial to patient outcome, for example by facilitating weaning [18].

In a study of twenty-five mechanically ventilated patients with severe COPD and systolic pressure variations 15 mm Hg, heliox was found to improve hemodynamics and pulmonary mechanics. During 30 min of mechanical ventilation with heliox, intrinsic PEEP, trapped lung volume, and systolic arterial pressure variations all decreased. In ten patients with pulmonary artery catheters, heliox decreased mean pulmonary arterial pressure, right atrial pressure, and pulmonary arterial occlusion pressure, and increased cardiac index [19].

Conclusion

Heliox has been used in mechanically ventilated patients with airway obstruction. It has been used with conventional ventilators, high frequency ventilators, and noninvasive ventilators. When used during weaning, it is associated with a 21% reduction in work of breathing by, by lowering the resistive component and is linked to lower intrinsic PEEP compared to conventional oxygen. Also, it is associated with a 15% reduction in respiratory rate, a 30% increase in tidal volume, a 13% increase in minute ventilation, and a 29% increase in maximum inspiratory flow. However, when administering heliox, careful monitoring of actual tidal volume and fraction of inspired oxygen is essential.

Key Messages

1. Helium-oxygen (HeO2) mixtures have low density and high kinematic viscosity, allowing for reduced airway resistance, alleviating dyspnea and improving gas exchange in patients with severe exacerbation of chronic obstructive lung disease or asthma.
2. Helium-oxygen mixtures can lower the work of breathing and the dynamic hyperinflation in COPD patients at the end of the weaning process, without affecting the breathing pattern by unloading the respiratory system by reducing the inspiratory resistances as well as the dynamic hyperinflation by acting on the expiratory resistances.
3. He/O_2 may prove useful in patients with high levels of PEEPi and work of breathing by unloading respiratory muscles, improving patient-ventilator synchrony and tolerance to spontaneous-assisted breathing, which in turn may be beneficial to patient outcome, for example by facilitating weaning.
4. When administering heliox, it is crucial to monitor actual tidal volume and fraction of inspired oxygen closely.

References

[1] Esteban A, Anzueto A, Frutos F, Alía I, Brochard L, Stewart TE, et al., Characteristics and outcomes in adult patients receiving mechanical ventilation: a 28-day international study. *JAMA* 2002; 287:345–55.

[2] Esteban A, Ferguson ND, Meade MO, Frutos-Vivar F, Apezteguia C, Brochard L, et al., Evolution of mechanical ventilation in response to clinical research. *Am J Respir Crit Care Med* 2008; 177:170–7.

[3] Brochard L, Rauss A, Benito S, et al., Comparison of three methods of gradual withdrawal from ventilatory support during weaning from mechanical ventilation. *Am J Respir Crit Care Med* 1994; 150:896–903..

[4] Thille AW, Harrois A, Schortgen F, Brun-Buisson C, Brochard L. Outcomes of extubation failure in medical intensive care unit patients. *Critical Care Medicine* 2011;39(12):2612-2618.

[5] Yang KL, Tobin MJ. A prospective study of indexes predicting the outcome of trials of weaning from mechanical ventilation. *N Engl J Med* 1991, May 23;324(21):1445-50.

[6] Boles J. M., Bion J., Connors A, Herridge M., Marsh B., Melote C., Pearl R., Silverman H., Stanchina M., Vieillard-Baron A., Welte T. Weaning from mechanical ventilation. *Eur Respir J* 2007; 29: 1033–1056.

[7] Proud, K. and others. (2020). Chapter 16: Ventilation discontinuance. In D. C. Shelledy, J. I. Peters (Eds.), *Mechanical ventilation* (3rd ed., pp. 637-666). Burlington, MA: Jones & Bartlett Learning.

[8] Jhou H-J, Chen P-H, Ou-Yang L-J, Lin C, Tang S-E, Lee C-H. Methods of weaning from mechanical ventilation in adult: a network meta-analysis. *Front Med (Lausanne)* 2021. doi:10.3389/fmed.2021.752984.

[9] Ouellette, D. R. and others. Liberation from mechanical ventilation in critically ill adults: An official American College of Chest Physicians/American Thoracic Society clinical practice guideline: Inspiratory pressure augmentation during spontaneous breathing trials, protocols minimizing sedation, and noninvasive ventilation at once after extubation. *Chest* 2017, 151(1), 166-180.

[10] Dubois A. Resistance to breathing. Handbook of Physiology. Edited by Macklem PT, Mead J. Bethesda: *American Society of Physiology* 1986. pp. 451–461.

[11] Kleiman, A. M., & Huffmyer, J. L. Helium: Is the Sky the Limit? *Respiratory Care* 2018. 63(4), 488–490.

[12] Eves ND, Ford GT. Helium-oxygen: A versatile therapy to "lighten the load" of chronic obstructive pulmonary disease. *Respir Med COPD Update* 2007; 3:87–94.

[13] Hashemian, S. M., & Fallahian, F. The use of heliox in critical care. *International Journal of Critical Illness & Injury Science* 2014. 4(2), 138–142.

[14] Ho LI, Harn HJ, Lien TC, Hu PY, Wang JH. Postextubation laryngeal edema in adults: risk factor evaluation and prevention by hydrocortisone. *Intensive Care Med* 1996, Sep;22(9):933-6.

[15] Jaber S., Fodil R., Carlucci A., et al.: Noninvasive Ventilation with Helium–Oxygen in Acute Exacerbations of Chronic Obstructive Pulmonary Disease. *Am J Respir Crit Care Med* 2000, 161. pp: 1191–1200.

[16] Diehl JL, Mercat A Guérot E, Aïssa F, Teboul JL, Richard C, Labrousse J Helium/oxygen mixture reduces the work of breathing at the end of the weaning process in patients with severe chronic obstructive pulmonary disease. *Crit Care Med* 2003. 31:1415–1420..

[17] Tatsuno K, Imai Y, Konno S. Therapeutic use of helium-oxygen mixture in continuous positive airway pressure for early weaning from mechanical ventilation after cardiovascular surgery in infants. *J Thorac Cardiovasc Surg* 1976. Jul;72(1):119-22.

[18] Tassaux D, Gainnier M, Battisti A, Jolliet P. Helium-oxygen decreases inspiratory effort and work of breathing during pressure support in intubated patients with chronic obstructive pulmonary disease. *Intensive Care Med* 2005, Nov;31(11):1501-7.

[19] Lee DL, Lee H, Chang HW, Chang AY, Lin SL, Huang YC. Heliox improves hemodynamics in mechanically ventilated patients with chronic obstructive pulmonary disease with systolic pressure variations. *Crit Care Med* 2005;33(5):968–97.

Chapter 18

Heliox Therapy in Tracheostomy

Selma Mine Kara Apaydın*, MD
Eskisehir City Hospital, Eskisehir, Turkey

Abstract

Heliox is a respiratory gas consisting of a mixture of helium and oxygen. It can be used as an adjunct in the treatment of severe airway obstruction due to its high CO_2 diffusion coefficient and fluidity. While it has no direct therapeutic effect, it serves as a temporary palliative measure until more definitive treatments take effect. Tracheostomy is indicated in intubated patients who are being monitored in the following situations:: inability to develop a weaning plan, failure of extubation, difficulty in weaning and prolonged dependency on respiratory support. In these cases, performing a tracheostomy is preferred between days 2 and 10. The optimal timing is controversial; however, recent studies have shown that performing a tracheostomy earlier than 14 dayscan shorten the length of stay in the intensive care unit. The reasons for performing an awake tracheostomy due to airway obstruction can be benign or malignant diseases. Benign conditions requiring awake tracheostomy include benign laryngeal tumors, subglottic stenosis, inflammatory conditions (such as deep neck infection and angioedema), bilateral vocal cord paralysis, maxillofacial trauma and burns. Either surgical or percutaneous tracheostomy methods can be used. The appropriate method should be determined according to hospital resources and the experience of the team planning the procedure.

---

* Corresponding Author's Email: md_selmika@hotmail.com

In: Respiratory Care in Heliox Therapy Physiology and Technology
Editor: Antonio M. Esquinas
ISBN: 979-8-89530-385-6

Keywords: tracheostomy, airway obstruction, respiratory diseases, intensive care unit, treatment strategies

Introduction

Tracheotomy, in its simplest definition, is the process of opening a path through the anterior wall of the trachea to create an adequate airway. Tracheostomy is the process of creating a stoma on the skin surface leading to the trachea. It is the oldest known life-saving respiratory method in the history of medicine, with applications documented in Egypt as early as 3600 BC [1]. Tracheostomy should be considered for all patients with airway obstruction or those at risk of a difficult intubation.

Tracheostomy is a surgical procedure that requires experience. Ideally, itshould be performed under general anesthesia after endotracheal intubation, although it can also be performed under local anesthesia in emergencies and in cases where intubation cannot be performed. The risk of serious complications during or after emergency tracheostomyncreases; therefore it is best performed before an emergency occurs.

Indications for Tracheostomy

1. Upper airway obstruction (e.g., tumors of upper trachea, infections such as epiglottitis, bilateral vocal cord paralysis, laryngeal or maxillofacial traumas, foreign body obstruction, subglottic tracheal stenosis)
2. Patients requiring long-term mechanical ventilation (e.g., endotracheal tube use for more than one week)
3. Conditions necessitating adequate clearance of bronchial secretions to maintain airway integrity
4. Elective procedures (e.g., before major head and neck surgeries) [2-3].

Conditions that may require tracheostomyinclude infective or malignant diseases of the larynx, trachea or oropharynx causing upper respiratory tract obstruction, foreign body aspiration, expected respiratory difficulty after surgery, maxillofacial/laryngeal/tracheal injuries, burns to the face/neck/upper respiratory tract, congenital anomalies, bilateral vocal cord paralysis, tracheobronchial secretion aspiration, chronic obstructive pulmonary disease/hypoventilation, post-intoxication respiratory depression, post-traumatic rib fractures and subcutaneous emphysema, and chest wall paralysis. In these and similar cases, the goal is to correct pulmonary ventilation dysfunction. As dyspnea progresses, contractions begin in the suprasternal, supraclavicular and intercostal muscle structures. Symptoms such as disorientation and cyanosis can occur due to carbon dioxide retention, with rising blood pressure leading to hypertension. Respiration function may weaken, potentially resulting in coma. There is no fixed rule for determining the timing of a tracheotomy. The physician monitoring acute pulmonary dysfunction decides when to proceed [4].

Before the procedure, preliminary preparations are made. Hemodynamic stability should be ensured and the procedure performed by an experienced team after ensuring that the FiO2 value is below 60%, the PEEP value is below 10 mmHg, the systemic infection is controlled, and anticoagulants have been discontinued. Informed consent must be obtained from the patient or the patient's relatives. Studies show that patients with better lung mechanics (lower PEEP value) have a higher chance of weaning from mechanical ventilation after tracheostomy [5].

Table 1. Types of tracheostomy

Types of Tracheostomy		Types of Tracheostomy Technique	Types of tracheostomy
Depending on site:	High Mid Low	Cricothyroidotomy	Plastic and metal
Depending on the cause:	Permanent Temporary	Open tracheostomy	Cuffed and uncuffed
Depending on the timing:	Elective/routine Emergency	Percutaneus procedure	Fenestrated and unfenestrated
			Single and double lumen

Tracheostomy Techniques

Tracheostomy techniques are designed to reduce the need for sedation, facilitate faster weaning, improve oral care and feeding, enhance patient communication, and facilitate airway management outside the intensive care unit. Complications can be categorized into early (perioperative) and late. Early complications may include hemorrhage (minor and major), iatrogenic airway trauma, unintended decannulation, subcutaneous emphysema, pneumothorax, hemothorax, stoma infection, hypoxia, loss of airway control and even death. Late complications can include granulation tissue development, tracheal stenosis, tracheomalacia, tracheo-innominate artery fistula, tracheo-esophageal fistula, pneumonia and aspiration [6] (Table 1 and Table 2).

Table 2. Tracheostomy complications

Early Complications	Late Complications
Bleeding	Tracheo-esophageal fistula
Emphysema	Tracheo-innominate artery fistula
Pneumothorax	Tracheal stenosis
Paratracheal placement/cannula length insufficiency/ventilation leak	Granuloma
Iatrogenic airway traumas	Pneumonia, tracheobronchitis
Unintended decannulation	Aspiration
Hypoxia	Tracheomalacia

Cricothyroidotomy

Cricothyroidotomy is a temporary procedure intended for use in emergencies when endotracheal intubation is not possible, typically lasting 3 to 5 days. Risks include the development of subglottic edema and tracheal stenosis. This procedure is not recommended for trauma patients with cricoid injuries or children under 11 years of age. Cricothyroidotomy involves making a 1 cm horizontal incision in the cricothyroid membrane, located in the space between the thyroid and cricoid cartilage, and placing a tubein this area [7].

Surgical Tracheostomy (Open Tracheostomy)

This procedure should be avoiding trauma to anatomical structures such as the thyroid and cricoid cartilages, suprasternal notch, thyroid isthmus, carotid sheaths and recurrent laryngeal nerve. If conditions permit, the procedure is performed in the operating room, otherwise it may be done at the bedside. The patient is positioned appropriately, and a good light source is used to ensure safe dissection with minimal complications. The patient is elevated in the supine position with the head slightly extended. Local anesthesia is applied and sterile conditions are established. A horizontal or vertical skin incision is made to dissect the skin and subcutaneous tissue and to access and exclude the strap muscles. After opening the tracheal fascia, the tracheal rings are counted from the cricoid cartilage and a tracheotomy is opened from the second or third tracheal ring [8].

After the intercartilaginous membrane incision between the tracheal rings, tracheal secretions are aspirated and a tracheostomy cannula is placed. A balloon is inflated with air until air leakage stops, and the ties passed from both sides of the cannula are adjusted and knotted according to the thickness of the patient's neck. The procedure is completed by applying an appropriate dressing around the tracheotomy incision.

Some authors recommend using bronchoscopy to guide the cannula placement during surgery to prevent misplacement and injuries to the trachea. [9, 10].

When tracheostomy is no longer needed, the incision can be closed surgically or left for secondary healing. In some cases, tracheostomy is permanent.

Percutaneous Tracheostomy

Percutaneous tracheostomy is a minimally invasive procedure in which the cannula is placed percutaneously through dilation instead of through a surgical opening.

Numerous studies have been published comparing percutaneous dilatational tracheotomy techniques with other surgical tracheotomies. This method is often preferred due to its ease and safety, with complication rates reported between 1-10%. Most complications related to percutaneous tracheostomy are associated with the technique and procedure and can often be prevented. The primary indication for tracheotomy in critically ill patients is prolonged mechanical ventilation as it mitigates the side effects of prolonged endotracheal intubation. This procedure is widely used because it increases patient comfort and facilitates the intensive care unit treatment process. Before the procedure, anesthesia is administered, and positive pressure mechanical ventilation with 100% oxygen is applied. The patient is in a flat supine position, with the head extended and support under the shoulders. The endotracheal tube balloon is deflated, the tube is pulled under the vocal cords, and then the tube balloon is re-inflated. Next, the second and third spaces of the tracheal cartilages are palpated, and local anesthesia is applied to the area to the treatment area. A horizontal incision (8-10 mm) is made with a scalpel, followed by the insertion of a guide wire into the tracheal lumen using a 14G needle [11]. An 8F dilator is then passed over the guide wire to expand the lumen. After removing the dilator is, forceps are used to expand the skin, subcutaneous tissue and trachea, allowing for the placement ofa size 7.5 or 8 tracheotomy tube is placed into the trachea.

During the first 24 hours post-procedure, close monitoring for complications is crucial. Complications can include early bleeding, subcutaneous emphysema, pneumothorax, and ventilation failure due to cannula placement. Spontaneous breathing trials are performed prior to decannulation, considering the patient's ability to cough, vital capacity, effective deep breathing, airway protection, and the status of tracheobronchial secretions [12].

Endoscopic imaging methods can be used to support the application of tracheostomy techniques. The advantages of endoscopic imaging include verification of the access site, prevention of postoperative wall damage, and prevention of accidental extubation. However, there are also disadvantages, such as decreased oxygenation secondary to decreased ventilation, the need for additional personnel, increased cost, and prolonged procedure time [13].

The percutaneous tracheostomy method is considered as an alternative to surgical tracheostomy. However, complications such as cuff perforation, extubation and aspiration may occur during the procedure. To reduce these complications, supraglottic airway devices such as the laryngeal mask can be used during the procedure. Anatomical variations of the neck structures can increase the risk of hemorrhage during percutaneous interventions. This risk is particularly heightened in patients with short necks, making the use of ultrasound guidance advisable to minimize the variations seen in the brachiocephalic veins and reduce the potential for hemorrhage during or after the procedure [14].

Tracheotomy Decannulation

A decannulation plan can be made for clinically stable patients who have a $PaCO_2$ less than 60 mmHg in arterial blood gas, no psychiatric disorders, no stenosis on bronchoscopic examination, and the ability to swallow and produce sputum adequately. After removing the tracheostomy tube, the wound can be sutured or dressed for secondary healing, with the stoma expected to heal spontaneously in approximately 10 days [15].

Results

In some cases, a delayed tracheotomy may be necessary, particularly in patients experiencing severe hypoxemia or bleeding diathesis. In addition, the hesitation of the patient or relatives to give consent for tracheotomy may cause the postponement of the procedure. In situations where disease progression is unpredictable, such as moderate cerebral damage, neuromuscular diseases, or moderate to severe chronic lung pathologies, the physician's decision-making period may extend for weeks. Patients without significant mortality risk can be discharged from intensive care units and sent to normal patient wards or to their homes with home-type mechanical ventilators.

Conclusion

Tracheotomy is recommended to avoid complications associated with prolonged intubation in patients requiring mechanical ventilation support. The procedure should be performed as soon as possible to expedite treatment and faciliate weaning from mechanical ventilation.

Key Messages

1. Early tracheotomy can reduce the rate of ventilator-associated pneumonia, positively impacting complications and hospitalization.
2. The physician overseeing the care determines the appropriate timing andmethod for tracheostomy.
3. Tracheostomy enhances the patient's comfort and participation in activites such as eating, speaking, and communicating.
4. Both surgical and percutaneous tracheostomy are viable options.
5. Permanent tracheostomies should not be avoided when clinically necessary.

References

[1] Lasala J. History of Airway Management. *Journal of Anesthesia History* 2015;1(3):96-7.

[2] MacIntyre NR, Cook DJ, Ely EW, et al., Evidence-based guidelines for weaning and discontinuing ventilatory support: a collective task force facilitated by the American College of Chest Physicians; the American Association for Respiratory Care and the American College of Critical Care Medicine. *Chest* 2001;120(6):375-95.

[3] Susaman N, Hanbeyoglu O. Comparıson between surgıcal and percutaneous tracheostomy effects on gerıatrıc patıents in the ICU. *Turkish Journal of Geriatrics* 2020;23:188-196.

[4] Freeman BD, Isabella K, Lin N, et al., A meta-analysis of prospective trials comparing percutaneous and surgical tracheostomy in critically ill patients. *Chest* 2000;118:1412-18.

[5] M C Lin, C C Huang, C T Yang, Y H Tsai, T C Tsao . Pulmonary Mechanics in Patients with Prolonged MechanicalVentilation Requiring Tracheostomy. *Anaesth Intensive Care* 1999; 27: 581-85.

[6] Grillo HC. Tracheostomy: uses, varieties, complications. Surgery of the trachea and bronchi. Hamilton, London: BC Decker Inc. 2004;10:291-300.

[7] Christina G Rehm, Sandra M Wanek, Eliot B Gagnon, Slone K Pearson and Richard J Mullins. Cricothyroidotomy for elective airway management in critically ill trauma patients with technically challenging neck anatomy. *Critical Care* 2002;6:531-35.

[8] Paul De Leyn, Lieven Bedert, Marion Delcroix, Pieter Depuydt, Geert Lauwers, Youri Sokolov et al., Tracheotomy: clinical review and guidelines. *European Journal of Cardio-thoracic Surgery* 2007; 32:412-21.

[9] Polderman, KH, Spijkstra JJ, de Bree R, Christiaans HM, Gelissen HP, Wester JP et al., Percutaneous dilatational tracheostomy in the ICU: optimal organization, low complication rates, and description of a new complication. *Chest* 2003; 123(5), 1595-1602.

[10] Romero CM, Cornejo RA, Ruiz MH, Gálvez LR, Llanos OP, Tobar EA et al., Fiberoptic bronchoscopy-assisted percutaneous tracheostomy is safe in obese critically ill patients: a prospective and comparative study. *J Crit Care* 2009; 24: 494-05.

[11] Griggs WM, Worthley LI, Gilligan JE, Thomas PD, Myburg JA. A simple percutaneous tracheostomy technique. *Surg Gynecol Obster* 1990;170(6):543-5.

[12] Boulos Toursarkissian, Thomas N. Zweng, Paul A. Kearney, Walter E. Pofahl, Steven B. Johnson, Donald E. Barker Percutaneous dilational tracheostomy: Report of 141 cases. *The Annals of Thoracic Surgery*, 1994;57(4):862-7.

[13] Lüsebrink E, Krogmann A, Tietz F, Riebisch M, Okrojek R, Peltz F et al., Percutaneous dilatational tracheotomy in high-risk ICU patients, *Ann Intensive Care* 2021;11:116.

[14] Raju K Puttaswamy. The use of Ultrasound prior to Percutaneous Dilational Tracheostomy. *British Journal of Anaesthesia* 2006;6:97.

[15] Christopher KL. Tracheostomy decannulation. *Respir Care* 2005;50:538-41.

Chapter 19

Heliox Therapy in Pediatric and Neonatal Patients

G. M. Schmölzer*, MD, PhD

Centre for the Studies of Asphyxia and Resuscitation. Neonatal Research Unit, Royal Alexandra Hospital, Edmonton, Alberta, Canada
Department of Pediatrics, University of Alberta, Edmonton, Alberta, Canada

Abstract

Heliox, a mixture of helium and oxygen, offers a compelling alternative to conventional air-oxygen blends for ventilatory support of neonatal and pediatric patients. Despite its first use in the 1930s and its documented beneficial effects, its widespread adoption remains limited. Heliox's unique physical properties, such as its lower density compared to air, allow for less turbulent airflow in the neonatal airway, potentially diminishing the work of breathing and improving ventilation. The gas's impact on gas diffusion, elucidated by Graham's law, further enhances oxygen and carbon dioxide exchange in the alveoli.

In clinical applications, studies have shown promising results in a variety of respiratory diseases. Heliox has the potential to decrease intubation rates and improve gas exchange in premature infants with respiratory distress syndrome (RDS). In meconium aspiration syndrome (MAS) there is evidence of improved oxygenation and reduced hospitalization with heliox but larger trials are warranted. In bronchopulmonary dysplasia (BPD), heliox exhibits potential benefits including lower intubation rates and reduced inflammatory markers. In bronchiolitis, while heliox shows promise in reducing respiratory distress scores, its overall impact on intubation rates and treatment duration is inconclusive

* Corresponding Author's Email: georg.schmoelzer@me.com

In: Respiratory Care in Heliox Therapy Physiology and Technology
Editor: Antonio M. Esquinas
ISBN: 979-8-89530-385-6

and requires further investigation. Safety concerns, such as the potential for hypothermia, emphasize the importance of careful monitoring during heliox therapy. While existing evidence suggests heliox's efficacy, larger, well-designed trials are essential to validate its widespread use in neonatal and pediatric ventilatory support.

Keywords: newborn infants, neonatal intensive care unit, pediatric intensive care unit, heliox

Introduction

Heliox, a mixture of helium and oxygen, is an alternative to air-oxygen during ventilatory support in newborn infants or pediatric patients. Heliox was first used in the pediatric population in the 1930s, however, it is not commonly used despite described beneficial effects in observational and small randomized trials [1]. Heliox has been examined in newborn infants and children with respiratory distress syndrome, meconium aspiration syndrome, bronchopulmonary dysplasia, and bronchiolitis.

Physical Properties

Heliox is an odorless, non-explosive, non-flammable gas. Its density is about 3 times lower than the density of air [1, 2, 3]. The newborn's airways, characterized by a small cross-sectional diameter, exhibit relatively high resistance compared to older patients, significantly impacting gas exchange. Substituting heliox for an air-oxygen mixture diminishes turbulent airflow in the airways, enabling the delivery of a specific volume at a lower pressure [2]. Therefore, heliox may reduce the work of breathing, potentially reduce lung barotrauma, and improve ventilation in newborns and infants with increased airway resistance. Graham's law elucidates another significant impact of heliox; the rate of gas diffusion is inversely proportional to the square root of its mass density. Consequently, employing a helium-oxygen mixture instead of air, while maintaining an unchanged oxygen concentration in the inspired mixture, can enhance the diffusion of oxygen and carbon dioxide in the alveoli [1, 4].

Physiological Effects of Heliox

There are no confirmed toxic effects of heliox on the human body. Long-term studies on newborn rabbits, maintained in specially designed heliox-filled incubators, reported no adverse effect of heliox on growth or other physiological parameters, however, the study did not examine long-term neurodevelopmental changes [1, 5].

Clinical Applications Of Heliox

Acute Respiratory Distress Syndrome

Respiratory distress syndrome (RDS) is a condition primarily affecting premature infants, characterized by insufficient production of surfactant in the lungs, leading to respiratory difficulty (Table 1). The lack of surfactant, a substance that helps keep the air sacs in the lungs open, results in an increased effort to breathe and potential complications in oxygen exchange [6].

An initial trial by Elleau et al., randomized 31 infants with RDS to being ventilated with either a helium-oxygen mixture or a nitrogen-oxygen mixture for a maximum of 8 days [7]. None of the infants received surfactant; however, two infants from each group were excluded due to a grade IV intraventricular hemorrhage and mortality before the third day of life. In the helium-oxygen group, infants required a lower inspired oxygen concentration, shorter duration of ventilation, had fewer deaths, and fewer cases of bronchopulmonary dysplasia [7]. Migliori et al., enrolled 10 preterm infants who were ventilated from birth, and various respiratory parameters were measured before and during heliox therapy [8]. Subjects exhibiting a greater than 20% decrease in peak inspiratory pressure after one hour of heliox therapy were extubated and transitioned to nasal bilevel positive airway pressure with heliox for the next 3 hours [8]. The results indicated significant improvements in peak inspiratory pressure, work of breathing, transcutaneous pressure of CO_2, transcutaneous pressure of O_2, and minute ventilation, leading to successful extubation in eight infants, although one required reintubation after 5 hours [8]. This study suggests, that heliox might reduce resistive work of breathing and ventilatory support requirements and improve gas exchange in preterm infants. A further trial randomized infants born between 28 and 32 weeks' gestation with RDS to either standard medical air (control group) or a 4:1 helium and oxygen mixture (heliox group) for the first 12 hours, followed by medical air until nasal continuous positive airway pressure (NCPAP) was no longer necessary [9]. The results demonstrated that NCPAP with heliox significantly reduced the risk of mechanical ventilation compared to NCPAP with medical air (14.8% vs. 45.8%), suggesting that heliox enhances the effectiveness of NCPAP in the treatment of RDS in premature infants [9]. Similarily, heliox non-invasive neurally adjusted ventilatory assist (NIV-NAVA) ventilation applied in neonates born at or below 32 weeks' gestation resulted in a prompt and significant decrease in electrical activity of the diaphragm (Edi), while all other parameters were stable throughout the study, and did not differ between Heliox and air-oxygen ventilation [10]. Li et al., randomized preterm infants under 37 weeks of gestation with a diagnosis of RDS to receive helium-oxygen (n=19, heliox:70% helium and 30% oxygen) or air-oxygen (n=17, airox) mixture during nasal intermittent positive pressure ventilation (NIPPV) for three hours followed by airox until NIPPV was no longer needed [11]. Heliox significantly reduced the mean (SD) duration of ventilation compared to airox with 39 (15) hours vs. 58 (25) hours with heliox vs. airox p = 0.02 [11].

Table 1. Potential diseases for clinical uses of heliox in newborns and children

Newborns	Children
• Postextubation subglottic edema	• Postextubation subglottic edema
• Subglottic stenosis	• Subglottic stenosis
• Laryngotracheomalacia	• Laryngotracheomalacia
• Vocal chord paralysis	• Vocal chord paralysis
• Respiratory distress syndrome	• Bronchiolitis
• Bronchopulmonary dysplasia	• Bronchial hyperreactivity
• Meconium aspiration syndrome	• Acute asthmatic crisis
• Congenital diaphragmatic hernia	• Laryngitis, epiglottitis, tracheitis
	• Inflammatory etiology

A 2016 systematic review and meta-analysis included two randomized trials and one quasi-randomized controlled trial including 123 preterm infants with RDS and reported that heliox significantly decreased the incidence of intubation (Relative Risk (RR): 0.42; 95% Confidence Interval (CI): 0.23 to 0.78), levels of $PaCO_2$ (MD: −9.61; 95% CI: −15.76 to −03.45), and surfactant administration (RR: 0.25; 95% CI: 0.10 to 0.61) compared with standard gas

[12]. The current limited evidence suggests that non-invasive ventilation with heliox decreases the incidence of intubation in preterm infants suffering from RDS and larger trials are needed to verify these beneficial effects.

Meconium Aspiration Syndrome

Meconium Aspiration Syndrome (MAS) is a condition in newborns where they inhale meconium, a thick, greenish substance, into their lungs during or around the time of birth, causing respiratory distress and potential complications such as pneumonia or airway blockage (Table 1). The presence of meconium in the airways can lead to inflammation and decreased lung function, including elevated pulmonary resistance and reduced lung compliance [13]. Furthermore, severe MAS may be complicated by persistent pulmonary hypertension of the newborn (PPHN) requiring inhaled nitric oxide (iNO) [13].

There is limited evidence regarding the use of heliox during MAS. An observational study reported that heliox during mechanical ventilation significantly enhances the oxygenation index and reduces the alveolar-arterial oxygen tension difference, although the observed increases in peak expiratory flow rate (PEFR) and decreases in partial pressure of carbon dioxide ($PaCO_2$) were not statistically significant [1]. A small randomized controlled trial assigned infants to either heliox for 6 hours followed by an air-oxygen mixed gas (n = 35, intervention) or air-oxygen mixed gas alone (n=36, control). This study reported that newborns ventilated with helium-oxygen exhibited significantly higher PaO_2/FiO_2 ratios, shorter time to extubation, and reduced length of hospitalization compared to the control group on air-oxygen [14]. Additionally, $PaCO_2$ was significantly lower at 2to 48 hours after the intervention, and markers of inflammation and myocardial injury showed significant decreases. Inflammation markers at 6 hours and myocardial injury markers at 24 hours were significantly decreased with heliox, including interleukin-6, interleukin-8, and tumor necrosis factor-a (all $p < 0.001$); C-reaction protein ($p = 0.012$); and creatine kinase ($p < 0.001$). There were no significant differences in pneumothorax rates or other complications [14]. While these data are reassuring, larger clinical trials are needed to confirm these results. Furthermore, the evidence that heliox might be used in combination with iNO during PPHN is limited to case reports involving a preterm infant and a case with a congenital diaphragmatic hernia [15, 16].

Bronchopulmonary Dysplasia

Bronchopulmonary dysplasia (BPD) is a chronic lung disease that primarily affects premature infants who have received mechanical ventilation and oxygen therapy for respiratory distress (Table 1). It is characterized by inflammation, scarring, and impaired development of the lungs [7, 14]. Heliox, when used during non-invasive or invasive ventilation, has been associated with lower rates of intubation, decreased concentrations of inflammatory markers, and reduced oxygen demand [7, 14], suggesting, that it might be a potential therapy to reduce rates of BPD.

Although the trial by Elleau et al., from 1993 reported lower inspired oxygen concentration, shorter duration of ventilation, and fewer cases of bronchopulmonary dysplasia (2/13 in the helium-oxygen mixture group vs. 7/14 in the nitrogen-oxygen mixture group) [7], the study was conducted prior to the routine use of antenatal corticosteroids and surfactant administration. Similarily, in 1983 Wolfson et al., reported that helium-oxygen mixtures (80:20 and 70:30) when administered to spontaneously breathing patients with BPD using face masks appear to have significant decreased work of breathing, suggesting reduced pulmonary resistance [17].

Furthermore, Szczapa et al., performed a cross over study in 15 preterm infants with BPD while on mechanical ventilation in a predefined sequence (mechanical ventilation initially with air–oxygen, followed by helium-oxygen, and then a return to air–oxygen) [18]. During helium–oxygen mechanical ventilation, tidal volume (mean(SD) 5.25(1.46) mL/kg at baseline vs. 6.87(2.82) and 7.06(3.06) mL/kg after 15 and 60 minutes of helium–oxygen; $p < 0.05$), dynamic compliance (mean(SD) 0.50(0.16) mL/cmH_2O at baseline vs. 0.65(0.19) and 0.68(0.22) mL/cmH_2O after 15 and 60 minutes of helium–oxygen ventilation; $p < 0.05$), and peak expiratory flow rate (mean(SD) 2.92(0.61) L/min at baseline vs. 3.60(0.92) and 3.65(0.94) L/min after 15 and 60 minutes of helium-oxygen; $p < 0.05$) increased significantly, while oxygenation improved, and the fraction of inspired oxygen significantly decreased (mean (SD) 0.54(0.14) at baseline vs. 0.27(0.06) after 60 minutes of helium-oxygen; $p < 0.05$). Furthermore, during helium-oxygen mechanical ventilation, there was a significant decrease in the oxygenation index (mean (SD) 8.31(2.78) at baseline vs. 5.18(1.61) and 3.06(1.21) after 15 and 60 minutes of helium-oxygen ventilation, and vs. 5.97(2.75) 60 minutes after returning to air–oxygen; $p < 0.05$) and in the alveolar–arterial oxygen tension difference, while the PaO_2/fraction of inspired oxygen ratio increased significantly. Noteworthy once ventilation with helium-oxygen was discontinued, the infants' respiratory function and oxygenation deteriorated, and supplemental oxygen requirements increased [18].

While these data are encouraging, other studies reported poor tolerance of helium-oxygen in BPD patients, including behavioural changes, decreased skin temperature, and hypoxia [19, 20]. Larger trials are needed to assess whether helium–oxygen can reduce or improve BPD, as the meta-analysis by Long et al., (two randomized trials and one quasi-randomized controlled trial including 123 preterm infants with RDS) did not report any difference in BPD [RR (95%CI) 0.81 [0.38–1.73] p = 0.25] [12].

Bronchiolitis

Bronchiolitis is a common respiratory infection that primarily affects the small airways, or bronchioles, in infants and young children. It is the leading reason for hospitalization in infants and can lead to respiratory insufficiency in more than 50% of those admitted to the pediatric intensive care unit (PICU) [3] (Table 1). Seven trials, involving 447 infants under 2 years of age with respiratory distress due to viral bronchiolitis, have been summarized in a Cochrane review [21]. All the children were recruited from a PICU (378 infants), except for one trial conducted in an emergency department (69 infants). All the children were younger than two years (with two trials involving infants under nine months and one trail involving infants under three months), and seven different protocols were used for inhalation therapy with heliox [21]. Overall, there was no significant reduction in the rate of intubation [RR (95%CI) 2.73 (0.96 to 7.75), four trials, 408 infants, low-quality evidence) in the PICU and no increase in the rate of discharge from the emergency department: RR 0.51 (95% CI 0.17 to 1.55), one trial, 69 infants, moderate quality evidence] [21]. There was no decrease in the length of treatment for respiratory distress: mean difference (MD) -0.19 days (95% CI -0.56 to 0.19, two trials, 320 infants, moderate quality evidence) [21]. In a subgroup of infants who were initially started on NCPAP because of severe respiratory distress, heliox therapy reduced the length of treatment: MD -0.76 days (95% CI-1.45 to -0.08, one trial, 21 infants, low-quality evidence) [21]. No adverse events related to heliox inhalation were reported [21].

The Cochrane review further reported that the addition of Heliox therapy may significantly reduce a clinical score evaluating respiratory distress in the first hour after starting treatment in infants with acute RSV bronchiolitis (a significantly lower mean clinical respiratory score compared to those treated with air or oxygen inhalation: MD -1.04 (95% CI -1.60 to -0.48, four trials, 138 infants, moderate quality evidence) [21]. However further studies are needed before this therapy can be introduced into routine clinical care.

Safety Concerns

Helium is associated with a high thermal conductivity, which can result in hypothermia in patients receiving a helium-oxygen mixture [20]. This highlights the importance of adequately monitoring the temperature of the gas as well as the patient during treatment.

Conclusion

Heliox emerges as a safe therapeutic option with potential advantages for infants, attributed to its respiratory effects and possibly cardio- and neuro-protective properties. Existing data suggest that this mixture might reduce the failure of non-invasive ventilation and mitigate the risk of lung injury during mechanical ventilation. Future studies and trials are warranted.

Key Messages

1. Heliox, a helium-oxygen mixture, offers an alternative to conventional air-oxygen ventilation for newborns and pediatric patients. Despite its early adoption in the 1930s and documented benefits in trials, its utilization remains limited, warranting exploration of its potential in various respiratory conditions.
2. Heliox, with its odorless and non-flammable nature, possesses physical properties advantageous in neonatal airways. Its lower density facilitates reduced turbulent airflow, potentially decreasing the work of breathing and lung barotrauma, and improving ventilation. Graham's law underscores its impact on enhanced gas diffusion, offering a unique avenue for optimizing gas exchange in infants.
3. Long-term studies reveal no confirmed toxic effects of helium-oxygen mixtures on the human body, offering reassurance regarding

its safety profile. However, the need for more extensive investigations—particularly focusing on long-term neurodevelopmental changes — underscores the importance of continued research.

4. Heliox exhibits promise in addressing diverse respiratory challenges. In respiratory distress syndrome (RDS), heliox demonstrates the potential to reduce intubation rates and improve gas exchange. Limited evidence in meconium aspiration syndrome (MAS) and bronchopulmonary dysplasia (BPD) suggests positive outcomes, but larger clinical trials are imperative. In bronchiolitis, heliox shows the potential to reduce respiratory distress scores, though further studies are needed to establish its routine clinical use.
5. Safety concerns, particularly regarding thermal conductivity and potential hypothermia, emphasize the importance of vigilant monitoring during treatment.

References

[1] Szczapa T, Kwapień P, Merritt TA. Neonatal Applications of Heliox: A Practical Review. *Front Pediatr* 2022. 10:855050.

[2] Hashemian SM, Fallahian F. The use of heliox in critical care. *Int J Crit Illn Inj Sci* 2014, 4:138–142.

[3] Martinón-Torres F. Noninvasive ventilation with helium-oxygen in children. *J Crit Care* 2012.27: 220.e1-220.e9.

[4] Frazier MD, Cheifetz IM The Role of Heliox in Paediatric Respiratory Disease. *Paediatr Respir Rev* 2010. 11:46–53.

[5] Singhaus CJ, Touch SM, Greenspan JS, Wolfson MR, Shaffer TH. A Prototype Infant Incubator for Heliox Therapy. *Biomed Instrum amp Technol* 2006. 40:150–163.

[6] Sweet DG, Carnielli V, Greisen G, Hallman M, Ozek E, Plavka R, Saugstad OD, Simeoni U, Speer CP, Vento M, Visser GHA, Halliday HL. European Consensus Guidelines on the Management of Respiratory Distress Syndrome - 2016 *Update. Neonatology* 2017. 111:107–125.

[7] Elleau C, Galperine R-I, Guenard H, Demarquez J-L. Helium-oxygen mixture in respiratory distress syndrome: A double-blind study. *J Pediatr* 1993, 122:132–136.

[8] Migliori C, Motta M, Angeli A, Chirico G. Nasal Bilevel vs. Continuous Positive Airway Pressure in Preterm Infants. *Pediatric Pulmonology* 2005. 40:426–430.

[9] Colnaghi M, Pierro M, Migliori C, Ciralli F, Matassa PG, Vendettuoli V, Mercadante D, Consonni D, Mosca F. Nasal Continuous Positive Airway Pressure With Heliox in Preterm Infants With Respiratory Distress Syndrome. *Pediatrics* 2012;129:e333–e338.

[10] Neumann-Klimasińska N, Merritt TA, Beck J, Miechowicz I, Szymankiewicz-Bręborowicz M, Szczapa T. Effects of heliox and non-invasive neurally adjusted ventilatory assist (NIV-NAVA) in preterm infants. *Sci Rep 2021*. 11:15778.

[11] Li X, Shen J, Zhao J, Tang S, Shi Y. Nasal intermittent positive pressure ventilation with heliox in premature infants with respiratory distress syndrome: A randomized controlled trial. *Indian Pediatr* 2014, 51:900–902.

[12] Long C, Li W, Wanwei L, Jie L, Yuan S. Noninvasive Ventilation with Heliox for Respiratory Distress Syndrome in Preterm Infant: A Systematic Review and Meta-Analysis. *Can Respir J*. 2016. 2016:9092871.

[13] Huang H-B, Zhu X-Y, Cheung P-Y. The evolution of approach in the resuscitation of neonates born with meconium-stained amniotic fluid: a tale of two countries, China and U.S.A., in the past 60 years]. Zhongguo Dang Dai Er Ke Za Zhi. *Chin J Contemp Pediatrics* 2023. 25:229–237.

[14] Ma J, Tang S, Shen L, Chen L, Li X, Li W, Wu L, Shi Y. A randomized single-center controlled trial of synchronized intermittent mandatory ventilation with heliox in newborn infants with meconium aspiration syndrome. *Pediatr Pulmonol* 2021. 56:2087–2093.

[15] Szczapa T, Gadzinowski J, Moczko J. Heliox augmented mechanical ventilation in the treatment of premature infants with respiratory distress syndrome. *Pol Gynaecol* 2014. 85:939–943.

[16] Wise AC, Boutin MA, Knodel EM, Proudfoot JA, Lane BP, Evans ML, Suttner DM, Kimball AL. Heliox Adjunct Therapy for Neonates With Congenital Diaphragmatic Hernia. *Respir Care 2018* 63:1147–1153.

[17] Wolfson MR, Bhutani VK, Shaffer TH, Bowen FW. Mechanics and energetics of breathing helium in infants with bronchopulmonary dysplasia. *J Pediatr* 1984.104:752–757.

[18] Szczapa T, Gadzinowski J, Moczko J, Merritt TA. Heliox for mechanically ventilated newborns with bronchopulmonary dysplasia. *Arch Dis Child - Fetal Neonatal* Ed 2014. 99:F128.

[19] Butt WW, Koren G, England S, Shear NH, Whyte H, Bryan CA, Swyer PR. Hypoxia associated with helium-oxygen therapy in neonates. *J Pediatr* 1985, 106:474–477.

[20] Gamarra E de, Moriette G, Farhat M, Walti H. Heliox® Tolerance in Spontaneously Breathing Neonates with Bronchopulmonary Dysplasia. *Neonatology* 1998. 74:193–199.

[21] Liet J, Ducruet T, Gupta V, Cambonie G. Heliox inhalation therapy for bronchiolitis in infants. *Cochrane Database Syst Rev* 2015:CD006915.

About the Editor

Antonio M. Esquinas MD, PhD, FCCP, FNIV

Director international school noninvasive mechanical ventilation, director Non-Invasive Ventilation College of Experts. Principal research and academic publications are related acute respiratory failure, noninvasive and invasive mechanical ventilation (weaning mechanical ventilation, COPD exacerbation, hypoxemic respiratory failure and acute cardiac diseases. Published 667 articles and 60 edited books related with mechanical ventilation and noninvasive mechanical ventilation in pulmonary and critical care.

Index

L

M

N

O

P

R

S

T

U

V

W